P9-DTF-280

DATE DUE

DE 1 6 06			

DEMCO 38-296

R.

Community-based distribution of contraceptives

A guide for programme managers

WORLD HEALTH ORGANIZATION
GENEVA
1995

Riverside Community College
Library
FEB '99
4800 Magnolia Avenue
Riverside, CA 92506

RG 137 .C626 1995

Community-based distribution
of contraceptives

WHO Library Cataloguing in Publication Data

Community-based distribution of contraceptives: a guide for programme managers.

1. Contraceptive agents – supply & distribution
2. Contraceptive devices – supply & distribution
3. Consumer participation 4. Marketing of health services – economics
5. Programme development

ISBN 92 4 154475 9   (NLM Classification: WP 630)

The World Health Organization welcomes requests for permission to reproduce or translate its publications, in part or in full. Applications and enquiries should be addressed to the Office of Publications, World Health Organization, Geneva, Switzerland, which will be glad to provide the latest information on any changes made to the text, plans for new editions, and reprints and translations already available.

© **World Health Organization 1995**

Publications of the World Health Organization enjoy copyright protection in accordance with the provisions of Protocol 2 of the Universal Copyright Convention. All rights reserved.

The designations employed and the presentation of the material in this publication do not imply the expression of any opinion whatsoever on the part of the Secretariat of the World Health Organization concerning the legal status of any country, territory, city or area or of its authorities, or concerning the delimitation of its frontiers or boundaries.

The mention of specific companies or of certain manufacturers' products does not imply that they are endorsed or recommended by the World Health Organization in preference to others of a similar nature that are not mentioned. Errors and omissions excepted, the names of proprietary products are distinguished by initial capital letters.

TYPESET IN INDIA
PRINTED IN ENGLAND

93/9813 Macmillan/Clays - 7500

Contents

Preface

Community-based distribution (CBD) is a strategy that relies on trained non-professional members of the community to provide health services directly to other members of the community. In the case of family planning, these services provide information and temporary contraceptive methods, usually the pill, condoms and other barrier methods. Other primary health care services may also be provided through CBD, including oral rehydration therapy and treatment for malaria.

CBD is frequently confused with another innovative strategy for distributing contraceptives called contraceptive social marketing (CSM). The main difference between the two strategies is that CSM operates through commercial channels, while CBD operates through community networks and non-professional personnel. In addition, the fees charged for contraceptives are usually higher in CSM programmes than in CBD programmes.

This book is intended for use by programme managers, administrators and service providers who are responsible for planning, implementing and evaluating CBD programmes. It shows how to develop a programme that is appropriate to the needs of the community, and how to ensure that it receives support from the public, as well as from the medical community.

Successful delivery of CBD services is essentially linked to the education of potential users, and hence this book includes specific recommendations on training of CBD personnel as well as on service delivery. Chapters on monitoring and evaluation and on issues of particular relevance to CBD are also included, along with several annexes that provide sample materials that can be adapted to local needs.

This guide is one of a series of technical publications on family planning that have been issued by the World Health Organization since 1976 (see inside back cover). It summarizes the knowledge and experience of experts in CBD from around the world, including a review group that met in Washington in December 1989.

Comments and queries on this publication should be addressed to: Maternal and Child Health and Family Planning, Division of Family Health, World Health Organization, 1211 Geneva 27, Switzerland.

Acknowledgements

The World Health Organization acknowledges the help of Dr D. Skipp, Dr D. Pedersen and Dr V. Jennings in the preparation of these guidelines.

Many valuable comments were received from a review group that met in Washington in December 1989. The participants were: Dr E. Aldaba-Lim, Philippines; Dr E. Boohene, Zimbabwe; Dr W. Budiharga, Indonesia; Ms M. Cabral, WHO, Geneva, Switzerland; Dr M. Urbina Fuentes, Mexico; Dr K. Gulhati, United States of America; Professor O. A. Ladipo, Nigeria; Dr A. Mechbal, Morocco; Dr L. Mehra, WHO, Geneva, Switzerland; Ms E. Monthereoso, Guatemala; Dr G. Perkins, The Program for Appropriate Technology in Health (PATH); Dr M. Potts, Family Health International; Mr K. Seshagiri Rao, Family Planning Association of India; Mr M. Schiavo, Sociedade Civil de Bem-Estar Familiar no Brazil (BEMFAM); Dr I. H. Shah, WHO, Geneva, Switzerland; Dr A. Solis, WHO Regional Office for the Americas, Washington, United States of America; Dr J. Spieler, United States Agency for International Development (USAID); Dr M. Trías, Asociación Pro-Bienestar de la Familia Colombiana (PROFAMILIA); Dr C. G. Vargas, Centro Medico Carmen de la Legua, Peru; and Dr M. Wahba, Family of the Future, Egypt.

The manuscript was also reviewed by the following people, whose contribution is gratefully acknowledged: Dr H. H. Akhtar, Bangladesh; Dr M. Belsey, WHO, Geneva, Switzerland; Dr G. Brown, The Population Council; Dr J. Donayre, United Nations Population Fund; Professor D. V. I. Fairweather, International Federation of Gynecology and Obstetrics; Dr E. O. Hassan, Egyptian Society of Obstetrics and Gynaecology; Dr R. Hatcher, United States of America; Dr M. J. Hirschfeld, WHO, Geneva, Switzerland; Dr C. Huezo, International Planned Parenthood Federation; Mr A. Keller, WHO, Geneva, Switzerland; Dr M. H. Khayat, WHO Regional Office for the Eastern

Mediterranean, Alexandria, Egypt; Ms D. Kowal, United States of America; Dr V. Kumar, India; Dr A. R. Maruping, Zimbabwe; Dr. S. Mehta, Indian Council of Medical Research; Dr C. Mhango, Regional Training Centre for Family Health, Mauritius; Dr W. C. Mwambazi, WHO Regional Office for Africa, Brazzaville, Congo; Dr N. V. K. Nair, WHO Regional Office for the Western Pacific, Manila, Philippines; Dr B. Nassah, Rwanda; Dr V. Neufeld, Canada; Dr B. Pande, WHO Regional Office for the Eastern Mediterranean, Alexandria, Egypt; Dr D. Pierotti, WHO Regional Office for Europe, Copenhagen, Denmark; Professor J. A. Pinotti, Brazil; Dr S. Plata, United States of America; Dr E. Ram, World Vision International; Professor S. S. Ratnam, Singapore; Dr H. Rejeb, WHO, Geneva, Switzerland; Professor A. Rosenfield, United States of America; Dr R. S. Sungkur, Mauritius Institute of Health; Dr M. Viravayda, Ministry of Public Health, Thailand; and Dr M. L. Zimmerman, United States of America.

Thanks are also due to the following institutions, for providing information about their experiences in implementing community-based distribution programmes: the Asociación de Profesionales para la Promoción de la Salud Materno-Infantíl (APROSAMI) of Peru; BEMFAM of Brazil; the Consejo Nacional de Población y Familia (CONAPOFA) of the Dominican Republic; Family of the Future (FOF) of Egypt; the Family Planning Association of India (FPAI) CBD Program in collaboration with Banaras Hindu University; the Family Planning Organization of the Philippines (FPOP); the Family Planning Program of the Mexican Ministry of Health; the Federación Mexicana de Asociaciónes Privadas de Planificación Familiar (FEMAP) of Mexico; the Indonesian Planned Parenthood Foundation (IPPF); the Instituto Peruano de Paternidad Responsable of Peru; the National Family Planning Council of Zimbabwe (ZNFPC); the Oyo State CBD Programme of Nigeria; the Planned Parenthood Federation of the Republic of Korea; and PROFAMILIA of Colombia.

The financial support of the United Nations Population Fund (UNFPA) is gratefully acknowledged.

Introduction

It is now universally accepted that family planning services are essential to promoting birth spacing to reduce maternal and infant mortality.

It has been estimated that if family planning services were more widely available, up to 42% of maternal deaths could be averted in developing countries; the mean proportion of maternal deaths that could be averted is 24% (Sai, 1986).

The world fertility survey (Sathar & Chidambaram, 1984) showed that use of family planning methods varied widely, from 69% in south-east Asia to 11% in Africa. The survey also revealed that approximately 300 million couples in the reproductive age range did not want more children, but were not using any method of contraception. These figures indicate a significant unmet need for family planning.

However, simply keeping up with demand at current levels will be a challenge. In 1990, the United Nations Population Fund (UNFPA, 1991) estimated that the fertility rate among women in the developing world was 3.8 births per woman and that the contraceptive prevalence rate (the proportion of married women of reproductive age who practise contraception) was 51%.

According to UNFPA projections, based on the current level of contraceptive prevalence, the number of family planning users will have increased by about 108 million by the end of the decade, owing to the growing numbers of women entering the reproductive age range each year. Moreover, if contraceptive prevalence were to be increased to 59% of married women of reproductive age, the number of family planning users would grow by 186 million by the year 2000 (UNFPA, 1991). Annex 1 provides the current UNFPA projections for the growth in both contraceptive acceptors and contraceptive supply requirements in developing countries between 1990 and 2000.

Clearly, family planning services must be significantly expanded to cope with this demand. In developing countries resources are often scarce and many of those in greatest need live in urban slums or rural areas without ready access to clinic-based health and family planning services. Community-based distribution (CBD) of contraceptives can be used to supplement other government and private family planning services to meet this challenge to make family planning more widely available. It involves providing information and family planning methods (usually the pill and barrier contraceptives) in community settings, basing these services on the needs and resources of the community.

In most CBD programmes, people for whom these methods are not suitable, or who wish to use another method, are referred to a family planning clinic or other health facility. CBD can be an important addition or alternative to clinic-based services. It is usually less costly than clinic services, easier for many people to reach, and available in a wider range of settings.

CBD exemplifies WHO's commitment to primary health care by making essential health care available to individuals and families in the community in an acceptable and affordable way and with their full participation.

The primary health care approach has evolved over the years, partly in the light of experience gained in basic health services throughout the world. However, it means more than simply extending basic health services. It has social and developmental dimensions and, if properly applied, should influence the way in which the rest of the health system functions.

Community-based distribution is also compatible with the trend, in many countries, towards the decentralization of health services and the involvement of the community in the provision and support of its own health services. CBD services have been operating for over 20 years, during which time many models have been developed and tested. By the mid-1980s, CBD services were available in more than 40 countries, largely in Asia and Latin America, but also in Africa and other continents (Fincanciogly, 1984). To date, most CBD programmes have been operated by nongovernmental organizations (NGOs), although public sector institutions are increasingly adopting this approach.

Policy-makers, health planners, and family planning providers have recognized that CBD can be a highly cost–

effective means of improving access to family planning services in remote communities. Furthermore, because the community is directly involved, the services are more likely to be accepted, and they can be integrated with existing health services.

The chapters that follow provide guidance for planning, implementing and evaluating CBD programmes. But first, it will be useful to define some of the terms that are used throughout the guidelines:

Clinic-based services: family planning services provided in a formal setting such as a hospital, clinic, health post or other medical facility. Such services can usually offer a more complete range of services than CBD distributors.

Distributor: a community worker who distributes contraceptives and information about family planning directly to the community. Distributors may also be known by other names, such as fieldworkers, educators, promoters, canvassers or depot-holders. While distributors are usually volunteers, in some programmes they may receive modest salaries or a proportion of the fees charged for contraceptives.

Supervisor: a community worker who supports and oversees the work of the distributors and provides the crucial administrative link between the central office and the field. Supervisors provide guidance and technical assistance to distributors, identify those in need of refresher training, and collect and analyse service data. They are also usually responsible for carrying out information and education campaigns in the community and maintaining links with influential community members and groups.

Information, education and communication (IEC) activities: activities designed to educate the community about family planning and its benefits and to inform potential users about the CBD programme, the services it offers, and the location of its distribution points. IEC activities require careful planning and many use information channels such as presentations, lectures, community events, group meetings, printed materials and the mass media (e.g. radio, newspapers and television). They are sometimes referred to as outreach activities.

Logistics: the process and systems that govern the procurement, transport, storage, distribution and management of products or commodities, such as contraceptives.

1. Understanding community-based distribution

This chapter highlights factors that may be used to identify communities in need of CBD services, as well as factors that are essential to the success of such services. The concept of CBD is explained and compared with that of contraceptive social marketing. A hypothetical CBD programme is presented to indicate the issues that affect CBD services. This is followed by a chart that illustrates the kinds of people who work as CBD distributors in programmes around the world.

Community-based distribution (CBD) can be a practical, cost–effective alternative to traditional clinic-based services for expanding access to family planning for underserved populations. Populations in need of CBD services can be identified by the following factors:

- Low prevalence of contraceptive use.

- Lack of awareness of family planning.

- Low use of existing family planning services.

- Located far from family planning clinics.

- Shortage of trained medical personnel.

- Lack of resources to expand clinic services.

- Presence of cultural barriers impeding attendance at clinics.

In many developing countries there are an average of 7000–10 000 people per physician, with similar ratios for nurses and nurse–midwives. Clearly, these health professionals cannot meet even the basic health needs of the population. To compound this problem, the majority of these professionals are located in urban areas and are concerned with health services that require comparatively sophisticated training and equipment (Rosenfield, 1986).

Therefore, clinic-based family planning services are unlikely to be available in many communities, particularly those in poor urban or rural areas. For these communities, CBD is often the only means of gaining access to family planning services. CBD services are also usually more cost–effective than clinic-based services. (For additional information about how to analyse the cost–effectiveness of family planning service-delivery strategies, see Reynolds & Gaspari, 1986 and PACT,[1] 1986).

However, CBD is not primarily a mechanism to save money, but rather an effective means of ensuring that people have access to a variety of primary health care services in the community. In addition, because the community is involved in the provision of the CBD services, those services are more likely to be accepted and used by the community members.

Thus, even when sufficient resources and facilities exist to support clinic-based services, CBD can be an effective strategy for making family planning services both more available and acceptable to underserved groups or communities in remote areas. Many people who do not regularly use health facilities may be much more receptive to community-based services. They may have difficulty reaching health facilities, or they may be unwilling to discuss personal matters such as family planning with health professionals.

CBD and contraceptive social marketing

CBD is frequently confused with another innovative strategy for contraceptive distribution, known as contraceptive social marketing (CSM). CSM aims to expand the availability of temporary contraceptives (primarily condoms and pills) by subsidizing their sale, without prescription, through existing commercial channels such as pharmacies, shops and street vendors. In this way, CSM caters for the *informed consumer*.

CBD, in contrast, relies largely on community networks and non-professional, non-commercial personnel for both the promotion and distribution of contraceptives at prices generally

---

[1]Private Agencies Cooperating Together.

lower than those found in CSM programmes. In CBD programmes, information and education are as important as the contraceptives. This kind of information is not usually available through commercial channels.

The differences between CBD and CSM are less obvious, however, when CBD programmes distribute contraceptives for a fee through commercial outlets such as small shops, hawkers, market traders and street vendors. In fact, many programmes contain elements of both strategies and several CBD programmes have shifted to CSM as they have expanded.

Factors affecting the success of CBD

Community-based distribution is based on three vital ingredients, all of which must be present if the programme is to be successful (Table 1):

—support from the sponsoring institution, the community, and the distributors;

—accessibility of the services;

—quality of the services.

Description of a hypothetical CBD programme

The following is a brief description of a hypothetical CBD programme, which is based on the experiences of various programmes from around the world and is intended to help summarize the main points of this chapter.

Background

The CBD programme was developed by a local nongovernmental organization involved in promoting child health and nutrition. Four years ago, the agency became aware that there was a very low prevalence of contraceptive use in the poor areas of the cities and rural areas. Interviews in these areas revealed that three problems were preventing contraceptive use:

1. A lack of knowledge about contraceptive methods.

2. Difficulty of access to methods and information owing to the absence of local family planning services, and the long distances to clinics.

Table 1. Factors affecting the success of CBD programmes

Support	Accessibility	Quality
Strong commitment of the sponsoring institution.	Services offered at popular locations.	Sponsoring institution adheres to standards and protocols for contraceptive distribution.
Participation of members of the community.	Dependable supply of contraceptive methods.	Adequate training for personnel.
Adequate numbers of dedicated distributors.	Travel time and cost required to reach service points kept to a minimum.	Users receive all the necessary information to permit them to make informed choices.
CBD is acceptable within legal, ethical and cultural norms.	Waiting time to receive services kept to a minimum.	Contraceptives are medically approved, have not reached their expiry dates, and are locally known and trusted.
Financial and material support from the sponsoring institution, the community, and donor agencies.	Services affordable to all potential users, including those on a low income.	Client–provider confidentiality is respected.
Plans in place to ensure the sustainability of the CBD programme.	Services provided in culturally acceptable settings.	A follow-up system exists to maintain contact with users.
	Referrals offered for other family planning services.	

3. Unwillingness of many women to seek such personal services from strangers in unfamiliar settings.

Involving the community

The agency worked with its own staff from the poor communities to identify local leaders and influential community members. Meetings were held in the community centres and the leaders' help was requested to identify local women to act as distributors of temporary contraceptive methods (Fig. 1). The community leaders were invited to join a committee set up to plan and advise the CBD programme.

Distributors were recruited from among housewives, shopkeepers, market vendors and traditional birth attendants. More than 300 volunteer distributors currently participate in the programme.

Coordinating with other agencies

Programme managers also met with local representatives of the Ministries of Health and Agriculture to coordinate the

Fig. 1. An outdoor meeting of community leaders and programme staff

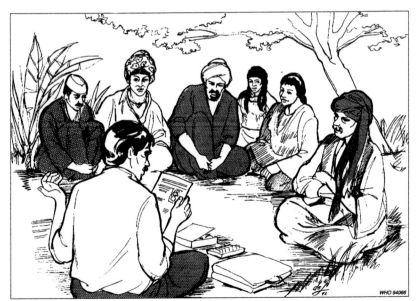

5

activities of the programme with those of the Ministries. The Ministry of Health (MOH) officials agreed to have rural MOH health posts provide medical back-up to the CBD distributors.

The Ministry of Agriculture (MOA) officials agreed to have agricultural extension workers carry family planning information materials and contraceptive supplies to isolated communities. They also agreed to coordinate their extension visits with those of the CBD programme, to allow supervisors to visit distributors in remote areas.

Training

Training for new distributors is carried out according to a strict schedule, and periodic refresher courses are arranged for existing staff in order to maintain the quality of the services offered. The programme recruits and trains new distributors periodically, to expand coverage and to replace distributors who have dropped out.

Providing services

The distributors offer pamphlets and information about the available contraceptive methods, counsel potential users to determine whether they have any contraindications to the use of certain methods, and help clients choose the most appropriate method. Table 2 shows the breakdown of services provided, by method, over one year.

Overcoming obstacles

The programme has encountered a variety of problems and obstacles since it started. The National Medical Association

Table 2. Breakdown of services provided by a hypothetical CBD programme, by method

Method	No. of users
Pills	2757 (47%)
Condoms	1812 (31%)
Foaming tablets	1010 (17%)
Referrals for intrauterine devices (IUDs)	290 (5%)
Total	5869

called for it to be halted, distributors left, and clients dropped out after an average of only three resupply visits. A women's association criticised the programme for "forcing family planning on uneducated, poor women". Fortunately, the programme director and her staff have sought creative solutions to these problems and now operate a successful programme, which enjoys widespread support and demand for its services.

First, the medical association was asked to participate in the CBD advisory committee to ensure that the distributors received adequate training. In addition, a contractual link was established with many of the association's members, which provided them with training in family planning, including IUD insertion, and a supply of low-cost contraceptives in return for medical back-up and referral services.

In addition, the medical association helped to persuade the government to modify the regulations that prevented the distribution of oral contraceptives without a prescription. As a result, the regulations now permit trained family planning workers to distribute contraceptives.

When distributors began to drop out soon after joining the programme, a survey was carried out, which revealed that the distributors' morale was low because of the hard work involved and the lack of financial incentives. After experimentation, it was found that distributors responded well to a profit-sharing scheme in which they kept 50% of the modest fees charged for contraceptives. They were also made eligible for promotion to supervisors, and award ceremonies and competitions were organized with good results.

However, the most successful source of motivation for the distributors has been a new training project in which distributors can register for instruction in subjects such as small business management, information, education and communication (IEC) skills, and public speaking. Besides enabling the distributors to set up small businesses, these new skills have also improved the quality of the programme.

High drop-out rates among clients led the programme to survey distributors and clients to determine how to improve the quality of its services. Staff discovered that clients were not familiar with the brand of oral contraceptives offered, disliked giving their names to the distributors, and were frustrated by frequent shortages of contraceptives.

In response, the programme changed its supplier to a local drug company producing a locally known brand of oral contraceptives. Client registration forms were modified to use only first names and client numbers, and the supply system was improved to ensure that distributors always have sufficient supplies on hand. The local purchase of pills also reduced the problem of supplies.

Finally, the women's association was invited to participate in the advisory committee and to help prepare appropriate information and educational materials to ensure that women are fully informed about all the contraceptive options. The programme is now well established and widely accepted, and is in the process of merging with the primary health care services operated by the Ministry of Health.

The above example illustrates the dynamic nature of a community-based programme. The programme began as a response to community need, and was then modified as necessary.

Examples of CBD distributors

Fig. 2 provides examples of the kinds of people who work as distributors in CBD programmes around the world.

Fig. 2. Examples of possible distributors

Market traders
Traditional birth attendants
Hawkers
Community health workers
Shopkeepers
Factory workers
Hairdressers and barbers
Traditional healers
Taxi drivers
Agricultural extension workers
Mothers
Farmers
Waiters and waitresses

---

2. Creating a foundation for community-based distribution

Regardless of the model chosen, every CBD programme must have the support of its sponsoring institution, the community which it serves, and any other groups or individuals whose opinions affect the programme and the demand for its services. This chapter identifies some of these groups, and outlines techniques for ensuring their support and cooperation. A method for estimating the potential demand for CBD services is also presented in a simple, step-by-step exercise.

Before beginning to plan a CBD programme, it is important to establish a firm foundation consisting of five elements:

1. Clearly defined placement of the programme within the organizational structure of the host organization.

2. Support from within the organization.

3. A thorough understanding of the needs of the community to be served.

4. Support from the members of that community.

5. Support from other organizations active in the community.

This broad foundation is not only necessary for starting the programme, but also for ensuring that it continues.

Placement of the programme within the organization

CBD is presented in these guidelines as a discrete activity to avoid confusion with other activities, and to emphasize its unique qualities. CBD programmes often operate in isolation from other activities within an organization, but even so, they must reflect and support the organization's overall service objectives.

The decision whether or not to integrate CBD activities within other service-delivery activities – or when to integrate them – is often made on practical grounds. In communities where other types of health care activities are already provided, it may be feasible to integrate CBD into those activities. In other communities where few, if any, health care services are available, it may be overambitious to consider introducing a fully integrated programme that includes CBD. Indeed, the absence of other health care services in a community is often the reason for introducing CBD.

CBD is frequently implemented as an independent activity by nongovernmental organizations involved in family planning. However, since family planning is a preventive health service, public sector CBD programmes are often located within maternal and child health and primary health care services, although functionally defined separate units may continue to exist.

CBD distributors often integrate other basic health services with their family planning activities. Similarly, CBD services may initially be integrated with maternal and child health services already provided through community-based volunteers. The degree of integration may vary from one location to another, and even over time, as the following examples illustrate:

1. Creation of a CBD sub-department within an existing division responsible for implementing a national family planning programme.

2. Introduction of a contraceptive distribution component to the existing primary health care services offered through community health workers.

3. Development of a CBD programme to provide a wide range of basic health services, including family planning, and operated by the maternal and child health care division.

4. Introduction of the principles of community-based distribution to various community-oriented activities such as agricultural extension services, adult literacy programmes, malaria eradication campaigns, and rural and community development efforts, but coordinated, monitored and evaluated by a central office in a separate institution.

5. Development of an integrated CBD and commercial retail sales programme that operates in conjunction with a network of family planning clinics managed by a nongovernmental organization.

Regardless of how the CBD programme is oriented within an organization, care must be taken to ensure that family planning is given the same priority as the curative, medically oriented activities. This can be largely accomplished during the initial planning stage by ensuring that the CBD programme has its own service-delivery objectives, workplans, budget, data collection tools, and reporting requirements.

Establishing support within the organization

Successful CBD programmes are those operated by organizations that recognize the value and importance of community-based family planning services. To assure support for the programme within the organization, programme managers should take the following steps.

Relate to organizational goals

Most organizations that already provide family planning or primary health services will find that community-based distribution is compatible with their organization's overall goals. These goals may include:

—improving the access of low-income citizens to basic health services;

—increasing the use of safe and effective family planning methods;

—addressing the needs of women;

—enhancing the effectiveness of child survival strategies in rural and poor urban areas.

However, in some cases, the organization may not have goals that can easily accommodate CBD. For example, the organization's goals may include:

—decreasing infant morbidity and mortality through the provision of neonatal intensive care services;

—providing immunizations and growth monitoring services to children of low-income mothers;

—increasing literacy levels in rural areas.

In these instances, the organization will need to examine its goals and possibly expand them to include CBD.

In all cases, support for the CBD programme within the organization will be greatly increased if it can be demonstrated that the programme will contribute to achieving the organization's goals.

Share information

As with any new initiative, it is important that colleagues are kept informed about the plans and activities of the programme. This will help them understand the CBD programme and increase their willingness to support it. Similarly, other divisions of the organization should also be informed about the programme and encouraged to support it through their various activities.

In addition, colleagues should be included in planning the programme. This may take many forms, from simply soliciting comments from co-workers, to asking them to review planning documents or actually participate in the planning process.

Win the support of health care professionals

The success of the CBD programme will depend on the attitudes expressed by the local health care providers. Health professionals, particularly physicians, can have a strong influence on the community's perceptions of the programme, the choice of contraceptive methods offered, and the distributors. Therefore, they must be convinced of the quality and efficacy of the CBD programme and its contraceptive methods.

One of the most common difficulties facing CBD programmes is the resistance of health professionals, particularly physicians, to the idea of delegating certain aspects of service delivery to non-professionals. For example, CBD requires that distributors are responsible for counselling, checking clients for contraindications to contraceptive use, dispensing temporary contraceptives, and making referrals for other methods or clinical services.

Health professionals are often apprehensive about allowing non-professionals to prescribe and dispense oral contraceptives without assistance from a physician or nurse. This problem can be overcome by ensuring that distributors are given adequate training and provided with checklists to use in screening clients for contraindications, and by informing physicians of the excellent safety record of CBD programmes. This topic is discussed further on page 85. (For additional information about the safety record of CBD programmes, see Serrano et al., 1987.)

Understanding community needs

Before setting out to win the support of the community, programme managers must decide where to introduce CBD services. To make this decision, they need to determine where the unmet need for family planning services is greatest.

Unmet need is defined as the number of fertile women at risk of pregnancy who do not wish to become pregnant, but are not using a modern method of contraception.

By determining the geographical location, the extent, and the characteristics of unmet need for family planning services, the programme manager will be better equipped to decide where to introduce services, and later, where services should be reduced or expanded. An assessment of unmet needs is an important management tool for the purposes of planning and allocation of resources. Furthermore, the assessment can be used as a basis for designing information and education activities.

Learning Point

A recent study in Zimbabwe highlights the importance of demographic data in programme planning. The 1989–90 Zimbabwe Service Availability Survey (ZSAS) revealed that the CBD programme was reaching a much greater proportion of women than previously believed: 76% versus 30% of women in rural areas. Although the programme had long been regarded as successful, because it was thought to cover only 30% of the population, the cost was considered too high. In the light of these findings, a decision was made to expand the programme. The findings also boosted morale among CBD distributors and other staff.

Information about levels of family planning use may be available from national censuses and demographic surveys (see Annex 2), or from special studies conducted at the regional or local level. It may also be available from service statistics maintained by the organization or other local service provider.

In addition, local health care providers and community leaders should be consulted, since they are usually aware of the family planning practices and needs of specific groups within the community.

Once the programme has been established, periodic surveys should be carried out to identify changes in the unmet need, and the demand for contraceptives. The surveys can also be used to evaluate the impact of the programme.

During the planning stage, a small-scale survey should be carried out to assess the demand for contraceptives and to identify any factors that limit their use. A model questionnaire for such a survey is provided in Annex 3. The survey should be repeated annually, or as necessary, to assess unmet need, to identify factors preventing contraceptive use, to measure levels of client satisfaction, and to determine patterns of continuation and method-switching.

However, not all women will be in need of family planning services. This may be because they are pregnant, breast-feeding, infertile, or because they do not wish to use a modern method, owing to concerns about safety, morality or other issues.

For planning purposes, a conservative approach is recommended that limits the definition of unmet need as "the percentage of fertile women at risk of pregnancy who do not wish to become pregnant, have the desired number of children, are not breast-feeding, and are not using any contraceptive method". This definition will be useful for determining where to introduce services, since it will identify the communities most in need of family planning services.

A second approach defines unmet need more broadly, as "all women who wish to limit or space their births, but who are not using an effective contraceptive method". This definition will be useful for designing an IEC campaign because it identifies, as far as possible, the number, characteristics and location of all potential users of modern contraceptives.

While there is no perfect formula for estimating unmet need for family planning in any given community, the following steps may be used to identify the communities most in need of services:

Fig. 3. Estimating the unmet need for family planning services

A. Total population in the community = 100 000
B. Percentage of women in the community = 49.2%
C. Number of women in the population (B × A) = 49 200
D. Percentage of women of fertile age (15–49 years) = 48%
E. Number of women of fertile age (D × C) = 23 616
F. Percentage of women of fertile age living in union = 74%
G. Number of women of fertile age living in union (F × E) = 17 476
H. Percentage of women of fertile age who are either pregnant, in-fertile, wishing to become pregnant within the year, or currently using a modern contraceptive method = 49%
I. Number of women of fertile age who are either pregnant, infertile, wishing to become pregnant within the year, or currently using a modern contraceptive method (H × G) = 8563
J. Estimated potential unmet need for family planning (G − I) = 8913

1. Begin with the estimated number of women in the population.

2. Subtract the number of women who are under 15 and over 49 years of age. (They are not usually in need of family planning services.)

3. Multiply the answer by 60%. (At any given time, approximately 40% of women of fertile age are not living in union, are pregnant, breast-feeding, or trying to become pregnant.)

4. Subtract the number of women who currently use a safe, effective method of family planning. The remaining number is an estimate of the unmet need for family planning.

These steps are explained in more detail in Fig. 3, based on a hypothetical community of 100 000 residents.

Choosing which clients to serve

It is unlikely that the programme will be able to reach all potential users of its services, even in a single community. In addition, there are usually different levels of unmet need among different groups. This suggests that programme managers may need to focus services initially on specific target groups rather than on the general population.

In most countries, family planning methods are less frequently used by rural populations than by people living in towns or cities. While this may be for a variety of reasons, such as differences in cultural values, education, or the availability of services, it indicates that rural areas are important sites for CBD.

In urban areas as well, there are often specific groups in which contraceptive use is particularly low. For example, recent immigrants, young people, and people living in poor urban areas may be appropriate target groups for CBD programmes. To identify these groups, programme managers should review relevant survey data and service statistics and consult local health workers and community leaders.

It is usually easy to identify communities that do not have adequate access to family planning services. For example, the *favelas* of Brazil, transmigrant communities of Indonesia, the refugee camps of Thailand, and the isolated rural communities of Zimbabwe all lack formal service facilities and benefit from CBD.

However, in some cases it will not be possible to extend services to the communities that seem to have the greatest need, because the organization will not have the resources necessary to reach isolated communities. The population may also be scattered over a large area, making supervision and distribution impractical.

Thus, constraints on resources often mean that a compromise must be made between the populations most in need and the ability to manage, supervise and supply programmes in those areas. For this reason, most CBD programmes are located in or near urban areas, or in rural zones that have relatively good transportation and communication systems.

Gaining support from the community

For the CBD programme to be successful, it must have the support of the community. As with other development efforts, the community must be involved in the planning and administration of the programme (Oakley, 1989). Such support takes many forms: labour; funding; materials; in-kind contributions and services; and help in identifying programme strategies, distributors and distribution points.

Community participation is important in several ways:

- Through participation in the planning and implementation of its own health services, the community is empowered by the knowledge that it can improve living conditions through its own actions, instead of waiting for services to be provided by external agencies.

- A community that is involved in a CBD programme is more likely to use and value its services, insist on high standards, and ensure its continuance.

- A community that participates in the provision of its own health services will be more interested in preventive care, including family planning.

- Distributors chosen with the community's help have the people's confidence. They often know the most effective techniques for promoting family planning among their neighbours and for winning community support for the programme. However, they must have a reliable source of supplies, as well as supervision and support.

Promoting community involvement

Programmes in countries throughout the world have found that involving key individuals from the community – health professionals, educators, political and religious leaders, and potential clients – in both the planning and implementation of the CBD programme is the most effective strategy for determining local needs and for winning the community's support. Most CBD programmes rely on community leaders for assistance in selecting distributors and many also invite community members to participate in the development of education materials appropriate to the local culture (see Chapter 4).

Since family planning affects women directly, women's groups such as marketing cooperatives, mothers' clubs, and women's training organizations can make valuable contributions to programme planning and can help to promote and endorse the new services. For example, in Ecuador and Peru, women's groups actively promote family planning.

Increasingly, mechanisms now exist at the local level in many communities that help channel community participation in support of family planning activities. Examples include: village people's councils in Burma; *jampinacuys* (community health discussion groups) in Peru; *sarailakas* (community-level economic development cooperatives) in the Philippines; and village health councils, committees, and community health workers in China, Thailand and elsewhere.

Learning Point

In Colombia, the family planning organization PROFAMILIA involves local shopkeepers both as advisers and as distributors of contraceptives.

In Egypt and the Sudan, family planning is promoted at the village level with the approval of Muslim *Imams*.

The Family Planning Association of India asks officials and influential village leaders to participate in the programme during the early stages. Officials and leaders are briefed about proposed activities, and are asked to suggest candidates for distributors (*raeda*). Some of them participate in the training of *raeda*, and they are invited to attend activities such as graduation ceremonies or public rallies. The programme also organizes 1-day training programmes for village leaders in order to generate support for the programme in the community.

In Liberia, tribal elders are consulted about and asked to help organize community efforts.

Similarly, in Nigeria, the Oyo State project seeks the advice of village leaders about which sites are most appropriate for CBD. These leaders are also involved in identifying potential distributors.

Whatever the strategy chosen for developing community involvement, the programme manager should:

- Learn and understand how decisions are made in the community and respect the local decision-making structure.

- Thoroughly understand exactly what it is that is being offered to the community. The programme manager must be able to explain to local leaders how their support for the programme will benefit the community.

- Be prepared for possible resistance among community leaders to the concept of the distribution of contraceptive methods and the provision of information about family planning by non-professionals.

- Be prepared to explain and discuss the health and social benefits associated with birth spacing. Programme managers should not assume that the community will see family planning as a need. Many communities place great value on having large families. In addition, some groups and individuals may perceive organized family planning as an attempt to control the growth and influence of their particular community.

- Explain to community leaders the many forms, other than financial, that community support can take. Often, people in low-income communities assume that they have little or nothing to contribute because they are poor.

- Be honest and open when dealing with local leaders and community members, and strive to establish a good reputation for services of consistent quality. It is very important to plan all the necessary support activities (including supervision, IEC, and the resupply of contraceptives, educational materials and service-record forms) carefully, to ensure that services are not interrupted.

- Keep community leaders and members informed of the activities and successes of the programme. Community leaders and groups should be consulted and included in planning any changes to the programme.

Communicating with other organizations

In many communities where CBD services may be established, there will be other organizations whose activities affect the health and well-being of the community. These may include the Ministry of Health, social services, private health and family planning organizations, women's groups, unions, businesses, and commercial groups or cooperatives.

Similarly, there are usually influential professional groups or associations such as international obstetrician–gynaecologists' or nurse–midwives' associations, whose support is crucial to the success of the programme.

It will be important to identify which of the above groups play an important role in the community in which the programme will be introduced. Communication with other agencies and groups is important for several reasons:

- The CBD programme can benefit from the ideas and experiences of other organizations.

19

- Other organizations may feel threatened by the introduction of a new programme. Communicating with them will help win their understanding and support.

- It will help to avoid situations in which other organizations are promoting conflicting messages, or are duplicating activities that could be performed more efficiently through collaboration.

- Resources such as information and materials can be shared, thereby reducing costs.

The first step in establishing links with another organization is to meet with a key individual from the organization, in order to identify areas of common interest. This will provide an opportunity to describe the programme's goals and discuss planned activities, as well as to lay the foundation for future collaboration.

The next step is to identify an appropriate liaison person within the other organization. Mechanisms that have been used by CBD programmes to maintain inter-agency communication include the exchange of newsletters, participation in meetings, health fairs, and other collaborative events.

By working with other organizations, programme managers will gain their support for the programme and be able to share their resources. For example, nongovernmental organizations involved in family planning may be willing to finance the programme during its early stages.

Learning Point

Nongovernmental organizations are frequently in a position to be more innovative than public sector organizations, and are therefore more able to adopt new approaches such as CBD. In Brazil, BEMFAM has collaborated successfully with state governments for many years. BEMFAM's approach is to establish agreements with local and state health officials in which BEMFAM assumes responsibility for setting up CBD programmes, training staff, and equipping clinics for medical referrals using public resources. The state or local Ministry of Health (MOH) administration then assumes responsibility for operating the programme, usually from existing health posts. BEMFAM continues to provide refresher training and supervision, on a contractual basis, to the local MOH offices.

Forming an advisory team

Once initial decisions such as where to initiate the programme and with which target groups have been made, an advisory team should be formed. Ideally, it should consist of key managers and service providers within the host organization, members of the target community, and other individuals whose experience may be useful.

There are several reasons for involving each of these groups. Key staff should participate in the advisory team because they will be familiar with the organization's goals, they may have experience working with the target community, and they probably will be required to provide medical back-up, training, supervision, or other assistance to the CBD programme. Including them in the advisory team ensures that their expertise is used and that their concerns are addressed early in the planning process.

Members of the target community can not only represent local needs but also serve as an effective, ongoing channel of communication with the community. Other people, ranging from community leaders to traditional birth attendants, may also be able to provide useful information about the community.

Health professionals, particularly physicians, obstetricians, nurse–midwives and nurses, should also be included in the advisory team to ensure that they support the programme.

The advisory team's initial role is to provide the programme manager with ideas, guidance and support in planning the programme. By convening regular meetings of the advisory team, encouraging a free flow of information and ideas, and incorporating the team's recommendations into programme plans, managers can substantially increase the members' support for the CBD programme and can benefit from their different experiences and perspectives.

The advisory team should also be involved in reviewing the programme periodically and whenever changes are planned, and in providing ongoing assistance in such areas as generating support from the community, and establishing and maintaining links with other groups and organizations.

3. Planning a CBD programme

The previous chapter described how to determine the extent of unmet need for family planning in the community. This chapter describes how to put the planning process into motion. It explains how: to determine how large an initial effort should be undertaken; to identify an effective community-based channel for delivering services; to set specific objectives for service delivery; to determine the numerous tasks and activities (and the timing of them) necessary to reach the objectives; and to quantify the tasks and activities in terms of the resources required.

Determining the scope of the programme

The previous chapter discussed how to identify where the programme's services are needed and assess the level of unmet need for family planning in those areas. The next step is to decide the scope or size of the programme, based on the resources available.

It is recommended that the initial effort be kept to an easily manageable size. Nearly all CBD programmes begin as small-scale projects, introducing services to a limited area to test acceptability and determine the most effective strategies. Once programme managers gain experience in providing community-based services in local settings, they may then combine the most successful elements of the pilot project to expand the programme to additional communities and areas.

If it appears that external financial support will be required for the programme, the programme manager should identify and contact international sources of funding. A representative from the donor agency or agencies should be included in the planning process. This will ensure that the sponsors understand the programme, and will be more committed to its continuance.

Selecting an effective service-delivery strategy

Devising an effective strategy or strategies for delivering services to the community is one of the most important aspects of the planning process. The possible avenues for delivering family planning services are limited only by the variety of ways in which the members of the community interact. The choice of strategy will determine how successful the programme is at reaching the community, how easy it is to manage, and how costly it is.

Distribution points

The programme manager should assess the most effective means of reaching the population. This will require knowledge of the community and how its members relate to one another. Mothers' clubs, markets, homes, shops, health posts, clinics, motels, maternity wards, beauty shops and community centres are all examples of distribution points with direct access to community residents (see Fig. 4).

Distributors

There are no limitations on the kinds of people that can succeed as distributors. They may be male or female, paid or volunteers, old or young, college graduates or illiterate. CBD programmes often have their own preferences, based on what is most effective and accepted in the local setting. For example, some agencies prefer distributors who work on the programme full time, while others prefer their distributors to work part time.

In Brazil, priestesses of *Candomble* temples distribute information about family planning, as well as contraceptives such as the pill, spermicidal foam and condoms. In the Dominican Republic, contraceptives are distributed through women's hairdressers in poor communities. In addition, prostitutes (male and female) in these countries provide condoms, as well as education and information aimed at reducing the spread of human immunodeficiency virus (HIV) infection and other sexually transmitted diseases.

In Egypt, Nigeria and Peru, men and women working in markets sell the pill and condoms. In addition, condoms are available from waiters in men's coffee houses in Egypt, and from barbers in India. Contraceptives are also available from women who make and sell herbal teas in Indonesia and from tax collectors and tortilla sellers in Mexico, while in Thailand, family planning services are available through taxi drivers and in floating markets.

In Nigeria, the Oyo State project has demonstrated that illiterate health workers can be trained to provide family planning services. The use of pictographs for instruction and labelling help to ensure proper treatment according to established protocols, and correct recording of service data.

In Egypt, Family of the Future has recruited and trained village barbers and religious leaders (*Imams*) as community outreach workers in order to encourage men to participate in family planning.

Fig. 4. Distribution channels
    (a) Home visits

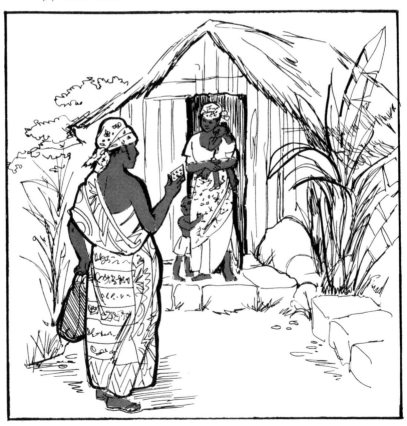

(b) Markets

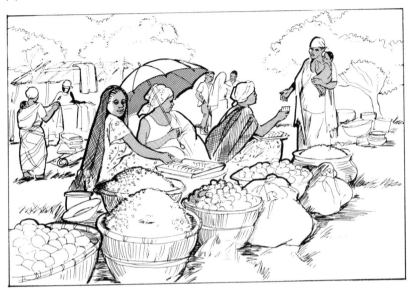

(c) Barbers

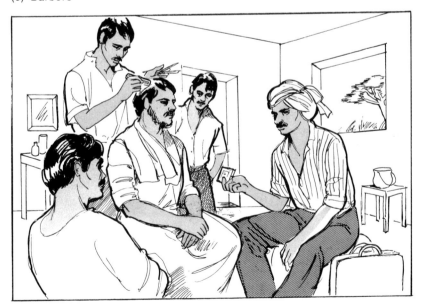

Despite the wide diversity of potential distributors, there are certain qualities that appear to be conducive to programme success in nearly all settings. It is generally accepted that the most consistently successful distributors are older, married women who are mothers, and are themselves practising family planning. Men appear to be particularly successful in promoting family planning among their peers and in distributing condoms.

Charging fees for services

All programmes must establish a policy regarding client fees for services. Until the early 1980s, few programmes charged fees for contraceptive services. Some agencies felt that it was not ethical to charge for services aimed at people on a low income, while others were constrained by official policies that prohibited fees being charged for public health services.

However, given the need to ensure sustainability of services, many programmes have now established fees for each service provided. These fees are modest and often linked to the prices for common, locally popular products such as cigarettes, beer or soft drinks. Many programmes have also established "sliding-fee scales" in which clients are charged according to their ability to pay. However, these have proven difficult to implement.

Experience has shown that a significant amount of programme costs may be recovered by charging fees for services, although it may be unrealistic to achieve sustainability through this practice. It has been found that communities place greater value on services and products when they have to pay for them. Implementing a fee system also requires that distributors are taught to maintain the accounts, which has been found to improve the quality of service data collection.

Once a programme decides to charge for its services, it must establish a pricing policy based on the clients' ability and willingness to pay. Some organizations require that prices are standardized and clearly posted by all distributors to ensure that services remain priced fairly for those most in need.

Other programmes have been successful in allowing distributors to charge whatever price they wish, provided that a nominal fee is returned to the supervisor. The rationale is that market traders and other distributors should be allowed to sell the contraceptives at the best prices they can get. This provides an incentive for the distributors and they probably know best at what point they will lose their sale.

Medical back-up

Adequate medical back-up is essential to all community-based programmes. Access to medical resources and supervision is necessary for several reasons:

1. To attend to family planning clients who require gynaecological or other medical services.

2. To provide clinical contraceptive methods, such as IUDs and voluntary sterilization.

3. To provide training and up-to-date, accurate information about contraception for CBD staff.

4. To ensure the quality and credibility of the programme.

Therefore, if medical back-up is not available from the organization providing CBD services, it must be arranged elsewhere.

Arranging reliable medical back-up is particularly important for CBD programmes that are part of organizations that do not provide medical services. An example of such a programme is the Maendeleo Ya Wanawake programme in Kenya, which is operated by a women's organization and receives medical back-up from the Ministry of Health.

Sources of medical back-up

Medical back-up may be provided at different levels within the national health system. In general, the more sophisticated or serious the need, the higher the level that will be required to provide the service. Similarly, medical back-up may be provided by a wide variety of health personnel, including physicians, nurses, nurse–midwives, auxiliary nurses and other health workers, depending on the nature of the need, resources, and local circumstances and norms.

Local health posts

Staff at local health posts can usually provide certain services for CBD programmes, such as pelvic examinations, Papanicolaou tests and primary health care. Some of these providers may be equipped and trained to insert intrauterine devices (IUDs) or even perform voluntary sterilization procedures. For services unavailable from these local providers, the user may be referred to a family planning clinic.

Family planning clinics

These are the ideal all-round source of medical back-up and technical assistance for CBD programmes. The staff are trained to provide clinical family planning services as well as certain other health services. Most family planning clinics are equipped to insert IUDs, many now offer injectables and a few offer implants. Many clinics are also well equipped to perform voluntary sterilization procedures. However, in the event of serious medical problems, chronic conditions or other major complications, the clinic will refer the client to a hospital.

Hospitals

Hospitals usually provide the highest level of medical back-up, and in many countries remain the only source of voluntary sterilization procedures.

Learning Point

As a result of operational research on medical back-up strategies in Peru, APROSAMI decided to set up local medical posts in the communities where CBD programmes are being carried out. Medical services are available at the posts 2 days per month and the dates are well publicized to the community. Each medical post covers an area of 5–8 blocks and is attended by a physician who, in addition to general medical services, provides advice on voluntary surgical contraception. The posts are open from 15:00 to 18:00. Patients with serious medical problems and those requiring voluntary surgical contraception services are referred to APROSAMI's central clinic.

APROSAMI has discovered that medical back-up is also useful in evaluating clients' knowledge of contraception, as well as that of distributors and local supervisors.

Developing objectives

Measurable objectives are critical to good planning in that they translate broad programme goals into plans of action that define what is to be accomplished, how it will be known whether it is being accomplished, and how long it will take.

Measurable objectives are especially important in the context of CBD where many kinds of personnel are involved, operating in dispersed locations with infrequent supervision. All staff members should have a clear understanding of what is expected of them and how their efforts contribute to the overall goals of the programme.

In addition, programme managers need clear indicators of their staff's performance. Measurable objectives will enable both staff and programme managers to monitor their progress and know when the desired results have been achieved.

The three essential characteristics of an objective are that it must be specific, measurable, and related to a specific period of time. An objective is acceptable only if it fulfils all these criteria.

This section discusses objectives that might be developed for a typical CBD programme. Basically, in a CBD programme the objective is to provide a particular kind(s) of service to a specified number of users over a given period of time.

To develop an objective for a CBD programme, the programme manager should start with a goal that expresses what the programme is trying to achieve. For example, the goal might be:

"To reduce infant mortality by providing families with the means and information they need to space their children."

This broad goal can be translated into action by developing an objective that contains the three essential elements:

Specific: "To establish a community-based distribution pilot project that will provide contraceptive services and information..."
Measurable: "to an estimated 4000 low-income women..."
Related to a specific time period: "over the course of one year (1993)."

Besides the essential elements discussed above, the objective may include two additional elements: quality and cost. Quality indicators are indicators of the effectiveness of the programme and might include the rate of continuation among users, or the percentage of users who experience an unplanned pregnancy.

While it is sometimes difficult to determine the rate of continuation among users, the level of satisfaction among clients can be used to assess the quality of the programme. The percentage of users who experience an unplanned pregnancy can reflect the effectiveness of the programme's counselling services and the reliability of the source of contraceptive supplies. However, this measure would require some form of additional data collection such as a local survey. Other examples of objectives that contain the required elements are provided below and may be used as models for programme planning.

Examples of objectives for a CBD programme

1. "To register 2380 family planning users by the end of 1993, by distributing temporary contraceptives and information to at least 8% of the women aged 15–49 years in three villages in the department of Libertad."

2. "To increase the prevalence of modern contraceptive use among women living in union from 17.5% to 24% by June 1993, by means of a community-based distribution project in the Matlab district."

Note: To form the above objectives, the programme manager must have access to basic demographic data concerning the age structure of the population and data on the prevalence of contraceptive use. This information may be derived from the national census, and community surveys of health, fertility or contraceptive prevalence.

3. "To register 2860 new family planning users and continue to provide contraceptive services and information to 2420 current users through 92 existing CBD posts, 30 new CBD posts, and a new programme of home visits, over 1 year, and at an annual cost of no more than 64 Mauritian rupees per user."

Note: The last objective introduces quality and cost indicators: the number of continuing (current) users and the annual cost per user.

Cost-limiting targets such as the cost per couple-year of protection can also be useful for improving programme efficiency. Such targets are normally set using only the "recurrent" or operating costs of the programme, and do not attempt to include the costs associated with setting up the programme.

Once the objectives have been set, workplans can be developed that describe the tasks and activities that will be necessary to achieve each objective. The activities can then be quantified in terms of the estimated cost of the resources required, and the budget can be drawn up for the programme.

Distributors

It is essential that each distributor understands what his or her personal service goal is, and how it relates and contributes to the overall objectives of the organization. Since distributors are usually volunteers, their main reward or incentive to continue is the satisfaction derived from knowing that they are contributing towards an important effort. Therefore, at the community level, objectives must be realistic and achievable, otherwise morale may decline and distributors will leave the programme.

However, personal goals vary widely with the skills, experience and drive of the individual distributor and with levels of demand. For instance, while most distributors will be capable of supplying contraceptives on a routine basis to, say, 40 users, there will be the occasional distributor who serves hundreds of regular users.

Furthermore, the personal goal may be expressed as a level of effort rather than as the number of users served. For example, each distributor may be allocated a particular area and be expected to visit a targeted number of households within that area over a specified time.

The setting of personal goals is done by the distributor and supervisor together. For further discussion of this procedure, see page 54.

Supervisors

Supervisors are the vital link between programme planners and actual service delivery. They should be assigned a component of the organization's overall service objective that they, in turn, break down and assign to individual distributors. Supervisors must have a clear understanding of exactly what is to be accomplished, otherwise they will not be able to provide guidance to distributors, or recognize unsatisfactory performance.

Once the programme is implemented, the objectives should be reviewed periodically. The objectives may have to be modified if they prove unrealistic or if circumstances change.

Developing a workplan

Workplans allow the programme manager: to define the activities to be carried out; to determine the time frame for each activity; to assign and balance staff responsibilities; to set personal goals for staff; and to develop clear job descriptions.

Workplan charts show each activity that goes into achieving a given objective, the time frame in which the activity will take place, and the staff resources required to carry it out. Some of the activities comprise "outputs", i.e. intermediate objectives that are measurable, but that in themselves do not represent the overall objective of the programme. This can be confusing since an activity such as "train 100 field workers" sounds like a measurable objective. It is, however, only one of several outputs needed to achieve the overall objective.

The advisory team, particularly those members from within the host organization, can be particularly helpful in developing workplans. During the planning stage, the programme manager should hold a meeting with them to identify each activity that will be needed to reach the objectives of the programme. To facilitate the discussion, each activity should be written down on large sheets of paper, a flipchart or a blackboard. A model workplan is contained in Annex 4 and may be referred to as a guide.

The programme manager should anticipate that there will be much revision and correction as the team thinks of activities to include and makes changes in those already included. As each activity is developed by the team, it should be written down and revised on a flipchart by the team leader, and then copied into the workplan. This should be a brainstorming session in which team members try to identify any possible tasks and activities that might be required. Therefore, all the suggestions should be written down. The following are important points for programme managers to remember:

- Determine every task, activity and step involved in setting up, carrying out, and evaluating the CBD programme.

- Determine the time frame for each activity, i.e. when and for how long each task will be carried out.

- Assign staff responsibilities for each activity. Note that many activities will require participation from staff at different levels.

- Once the workplans have been finalized, use them to develop or modify job descriptions for all staff involved in the programme.

- Finally, review the plans to determine whether any changes will be required in the structure of the organization. If so, draw up a new organizational chart and distribute it to all staff.

The completed workplan charts should be copied and distributed to all supervisory staff for review. Programme managers should be prepared for suggestions and review them with the team for possible inclusion in the final workplans. The charts should then be used as a guide during the implementation of the programme.

Identifying necessary resources

While it is generally recognized that CBD is a cost-effective approach to delivering family planning services – particularly compared with clinic-based delivery – a variety of resources are required to operate CBD programmes.

This section discusses resources that may be available from within the host organization, as well as resources that may be available in the community or from international funding agencies. This is followed by a description of how to prepare a budget for the programme.

Planning for sustainability

It is important for the programme manager to plan for the long-term sustainability of the new programme. Sustainability means that the programme can continue to function with only resources from within the organization (internal resources) and from the community it serves. Planning for increased sustainability requires that an effort be made on two fronts: cost reduction and income generation.

First, by monitoring and analysing the programme costs in relation to the services provided, the manager can explore ways to improve the efficiency of the programme in terms of the cost per user (or per couple). This will enable the programme manager to reduce the budget while serving the same number of clients as before, or to expand the programme to serve more clients without significantly increasing the budget.

Secondly, cost-recovery strategies can be implemented that generate income for the programme. Of course, the less it costs for each client served, the easier it becomes to sustain the programme through cost-recovery activities. Nearly every CBD programme operating in the world today pursues at least one income-generating activity. Possible strategies include campaigns to attract local donations (both in-kind and financial support), fee-for-service policies, and semi-commercial ventures.

This does not mean that self-sufficiency is easy or even possible to achieve, or that organizations, particularly not-for-profit organizations, can expect to reduce costs or increase income sufficiently to be able to do without financial assistance. Programme budgets, particularly for CBD programmes where the majority of staff are volunteers, are often difficult to reduce significantly. Also, the greatest level of unmet need is among people on very low incomes who cannot afford to pay prices that approach true programme costs.

Nevertheless, through a combination of improved cost–effectiveness and cost-recovery activities, many organizations are able to ensure programme continuity in spite of political and economic turmoil or reductions in one or other source of funding. Most importantly, the greater the degree of self-sufficiency, the freer the programme is to make decisions.

As a general rule, programme managers seeking financial support for the programme should first look within their own organization and then to local sources of in-kind and financial contributions. International sources of funding should be contacted only as a last resort. This will encourage managers to seek the most efficient means of accomplishing programme goals.

Learning Point

A wide range of income-generating activities have been organized by the distributors and coordinators in the Perkumpulan Keluarga Berencana Indonesia (PKPM) CBD programme. The strategies have included holding small lotteries called "arisans", and producing soya-beans in collective gardens (see Fig. 5) and raising chickens and goats. Many of the activities have been started with capital provided by the programme or the National Family Planning Coordinating Board, or with small parcels of land provided by the local Transmigration Department office.

Internal resources

CBD programmes can often use many of the host organization's resources to improve the quality and effectiveness of

Fig. 5. Distributors and coordinators working in collective gardens in Indonesia

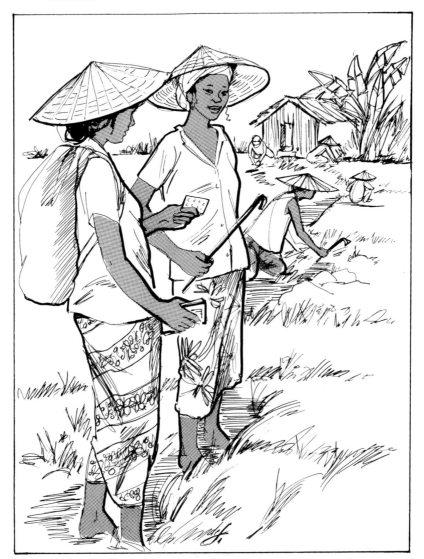

community-based services. For example, most organizations that provide health or family planning services have a supervision system which could be expanded to include supervision of distributors. Similarly, those organizations that have a

35

training unit may provide training for distributors as well as for other programme staff, such as supervisors and health professionals.

For example, when the family planning organization APROFAM in Guatemala decided to add a CBD component to existing clinic-based family planning services, the training unit developed a course for the newly hired CBD personnel to provide them with the basic information they needed to carry out their work. This required adaptation of the curriculum used to train clinic staff, focusing on outreach and communication skills, as well as on the specific tasks of the distributors. The training unit also incorporated CBD into their training programme for other staff of the organization.

Most organizations have a system for ordering, maintaining and managing the flow of supplies. In the case of family planning programmes, such systems ensure an adequate supply of contraceptives. Community-based programmes may require more supplies than clinic-based services and have different logistic requirements for distribution (see page 79). If the host organization has an existing logistics system, however, it can be adapted to meet the needs of the CBD programme.

The communications staff of the organization may also be able to assist with the CBD programme. They can include information about the programme in other organizational materials; assist in adapting, developing and testing educational materials appropriate for the CBD programme; and work with the CBD staff to design effective outreach strategies. In addition, communications staff play an important role in generating an organizational identity for the distributors in the community, which helps to create confidence in the CBD services.

The statistics division can assist by designing data collection forms appropriate to the CBD programme and incorporating the data into the organization's overall statistical system. There may also be other organizational staff who can be deployed in the programme, e.g. financial advisers, directors, and engineers (to maintain vehicles).

External resources

While the resources needed to provide CBD services will depend largely on the service-delivery model to be implemented, it is important to consider the resources that will be required from external sources. In most programmes, these will include:

- Contraceptives.

- Facilities and medical back-up.

- Financial support.

- Technical cooperation.

- Educational materials.

- Transportation.

Contraceptives

Contraceptives may be obtained from many sources. Various international organizations provide contraceptives free of charge to family planning programmes. The addresses of these organizations are listed in Annex 5. Some family planning programmes purchase contraceptives locally from pharmaceutical companies or other commercial outlets. This may be feasible, provided that the local manufacturers are reliable, and the cost of the contraceptives is within the programme's budget.

The important points to consider are whether an appropriate mix of contraceptive methods can be readily obtained (either free of charge or at a reasonable price), and whether the reliability of the source(s) of contraceptives is adequate to ensure constant quality and availability. If the kinds of contraceptives are limited, their quality is not consistent with clients' expectations, or their availability is sporadic, the credibility of the programme will suffer and clients will drop out.

Facilities and medical back-up

In nearly all CBD programmes, the community, public sector organizations and businesses help with donated space to house CBD distributors, store contraceptive supplies, or hold meetings.

Medical back-up may also need to be arranged from sources external to the organization. Private clinics and physicians are often willing to provide services to users referred by distributors, provided that they can charge a modest fee or receive free contraceptives. IUDs and kits for voluntary sterilization procedures are particularly popular with private physicians and can be traded for medical back-up services. Public and private health professionals will also support the programme in order to qualify for special training programmes in family planning the organization may be able to offer.

Financial support

External sources of financial support include donations from local private organizations, and contributions from international funding agencies. Although local companies generally prefer to make in-kind contributions of supplies, equipment and services, some also provide money.

Technical cooperation

Most CBD programmes have benefited from technical assistance provided by individuals with expertise in such areas as programme development and management, communications and outreach, and training. Ideally, this assistance will be provided by experts who have experience in community-based distribution as well as technical expertise in specific areas.

Several international sources of technical assistance are available to help programme managers plan their CBD programmes, design logistics systems, develop and conduct training, design and implement community-based activities and educational and community outreach strategies, and monitor and evaluate the programme. The addresses of these sources are listed in Annex 6.

Local sources of technical assistance should also be explored. Besides the sources considered above, technical assistance may also be available from the local university faculty, particularly the departments of sociology, management and statistics; the government statistical office; and management consulting firms.

The programme manager should carefully determine the kinds of technical assistance needed, identify appropriate sources, and establish contact with any potential sources of assistance.

Educational materials

Local artists are frequently willing to develop promotional materials, especially posters, that provide them with the opportunity to display their work in public places. Printing firms may offer significant discounts for producing materials on family planning. Similarly, discounts may be available for advertising the programme on radio.

Materials to support IEC activities are available from a variety of international organizations. The addresses of these organizations are given in Annex 7. In addition, many family planning programmes are willing to share materials they have developed. However, if programme managers use IEC materials from other countries, or even from other regions within their own country, they should pre-test them with the target audience, to ensure that they are locally acceptable and culturally appropriate, and then adapt the materials accordingly, before distributing them more widely.

Transport

Transport is often in short supply, especially for the large numbers of supervisors and distributors who must make their rounds. In some programmes, private bus and road haulage companies carry contraceptives and other supplies, free of charge, to isolated service sites.

Vehicles are sometimes available from international donor agencies. If such a donation is being considered, there are several issues to plan for. First, the programme manager must determine whether the agency will allow the organization to choose an appropriate vehicle. Unfortunately, many donor agencies restrict the kinds of vehicles they provide, consequently, those available are often not well suited to the recipients' needs.

In such cases, the costs associated with high petrol consumption, difficulty in obtaining parts, lack of durability, lengthy waits for repair, and insufficient carrying capacity can prove greater than the cost of purchasing a vehicle locally. If the potential supplier does not offer a vehicle appropriate to the programme's needs, the programme manager should ask about alternatives. Some donor agencies occasionally grant waivers that permit a wider choice of vehicles. However, many CBD programmes have found that other forms of transport are cheaper and more practical than standard motor vehicles. For example, bicycles (most popular), motor cycles, boats and horses are widely used. Use of public transport is also very common. The Nirodh programme in India and the CBD programme in Brazil share transport provided by other agencies. In Morocco and Thailand, CBD supervisors use mopeds and motor cycles. BEMFAM of Brazil, one of the largest CBD programmes, owns only two vehicles, relying instead on vehicles provided by the state governments.

Preparing a budget

Once the objectives and workplans of the programme have been developed, they need to be quantified in terms of the resources required and the costs associated with those resources. Annex 8 contains a model budget for a hypothetical CBD programme and blank budget forms for preparing a budget. It should be noted that the model budget is intended only as a general guide and is not suggested as an actual budget for the programme. The blank budget planning forms may be copied and distributed to the members of the advisory team involved in preparing the budget.

Since it is assumed that the team will have had prior experience in budgeting, and that the organization has its own budget format and protocols, this discussion will focus on those elements of budgeting that will have a direct bearing on the success of a CBD programme.

The budget should include the costs associated with each activity contained in the workplan chart. Resources that will be donated to the programme (such as contraceptives, space for CBD posts, printed materials, or supplies and equipment), or the equivalent costs of any volunteer workers, should not be included. However, it is recommended that records be kept of all the resources donated to the programme, since this information will be needed to analyse the cost–effectiveness of the programme.

The composition of the costs of CBD programmes differs from that of other programmes in that the major costs are usually incurred in three categories: training; supervision; and travel and transport.

CBD programmes require fewer physicians or other health professionals than clinic-based programmes, and only modest outlays for equipment, supplies, rent and utilities. However, CBD programmes can prove costly if the right balance of expenditures is not budgeted for from the start.

Training

The costs associated with supervision and training usually account for the largest share of the budget. However, if the supervisory and distribution staff do not receive adequate training initially, more supervision will be required to ensure that their performance is acceptable.

Furthermore, refresher training will become necessary much sooner, and for a larger proportion of the staff, than would be the case had the initial training been more thorough. Therefore, programme managers must ensure that the budget for training is sufficient, otherwise the costs of the programme may escalate in the medium and long term.

Supervision

Similarly, the budget for supervisory staff must be adequate. Supervisors must be able to spend enough time with distributors to observe them dealing with users, to review their records, to resupply them with supplies, and to provide guidance and support. This means that the number of distributors per supervisor, and the distances between each distributor must be considered carefully when the number of supervisors that will be required is determined.

Travel and transport

Vehicles may be needed for providing support, particularly in rural areas. Supervisory visits by central office personnel, delivery of supplies to distributors, and other such tasks sometimes require access to motor vehicles. If vehicles are available to the CBD programme, programme managers must budget for operating costs, including costs for fuel, maintenance, and repairs.

If vehicles are not available, supervisors and distributors (if the distributors will make home visits or visit the central clinic) must have adequate allowances for public transport.

Sufficient travel money encourages supervisors to visit more distributors, more frequently, gives them a sense of being valued and trusted, and greatly enhances their job satisfaction. Similarly, distributors are likely to visit more clients if they do not have to pay for their own transport. The procedures involved in providing or reimbursing supervisors and distributors with travel money should be kept to a minimum.

Other direct costs

Designing and printing. Data collection forms must be designed for supervisors and distributors, tested and then printed in quantities sufficient to the programme's needs. For newly designed forms, programme managers should budget for one year's supply, but only print enough for four months. This will allow the forms to be modified after three months.

CBD programmes will also require information and educational materials to be used at the community level. These

41

materials will need to be designed for the users, taking into account their level of literacy, cultural factors, and other considerations. This means that they will have to be designed by people with local experience, tested in the community, modified as necessary, and then printed and distributed.

Accessories for distributors. Programme managers should also budget for items that will help identify distributors to the community, and give them a sense of organizational identity. Such items may include briefcases or bags with the organization's symbol embossed on them, raincoats or laboratory coats, or signs to identify the location of the distribution posts. They can help motivate distributors, improve team spirit and increase public awareness of the programme in the community.

4. Implementing the programme

This chapter describes how to implement the activities outlined in the previous chapter. First, the process of task analysis is explained, to enable the programme manager to determine the personnel qualities and skills that the programme will require, and then guidance is given in selecting and training staff. This is followed by a discussion of the three vital elements that support the service-delivery effort: supervision; information, education and communication (IEC); and contraceptive supply.

Task analysis

Before selecting and training staff for each level of the programme, programme managers should first examine the specific tasks that each will be expected to accomplish.

Analysing these tasks will help the manager to determine:

- What skills are needed to carry out each task.

- What qualifications are needed for staff at each level.

- How much time each task will require (see page 31).

- Whether additional staff will be needed.

- What kinds of training will be needed.

Task analysis provides the basis for developing job descriptions for staff at each level. This is an important step. Job descriptions help programme managers to select staff, and to decide the kinds of training and supervision needed. Job descriptions are also useful to staff as a guide and reminder of their responsibilities.

The following are examples of tasks performed by staff at each level of a CBD programme. The specific tasks will vary according to the circumstances of each programme.

Central staff

Central staff are responsible for policy-making, strategic planning, administration, and the allocation of resources. Examples of central staff responsible for these tasks may include executive directors, administrators, the chief of the programme, information and communications officers, and financial administrative officers. In some organizations several individuals perform these tasks, while in others one person will be responsible. Their tasks include:

1. Setting the goals and objectives of the programme.
2. Developing strategies for achieving the goals and objectives and allocating resources accordingly.
3. Arranging for the procurement of contraceptives and other supplies.
4. Determining whether supervisory staff will deliver contraceptive services such as IUD insertion.
5. Providing technical support such as training, evaluation, and accounting, as required.
6. Coordinating training with staff at the intermediate and local level. Developing training guidelines for trainers.
7. Analysing service and financial data on a regular basis to determine the need for changes in the programme or its objectives.
8. Holding regular meetings with intermediate-level staff to discuss and coordinate programme activities and results.
9. Communicating regularly with all staff and with other agencies regarding the results of the programme and its contribution to the organization's goals.
10. Coordinating financial accounting procedures with staff.
11. Monitoring the finances and progress of the programme and preparing regular reports.
12. Monitoring the performance of staff at the intermediate and local level and providing feedback.

Supervisory staff

Supervisory staff are primarily responsible for supervision, training, making contact with the community and promotion. In decentralized programmes, staff may need to adapt strategies to local conditions in order to accomplish the goals and objectives of the programme. Examples of supervisory staff responsible for these functions include trainers, regional and local supervisors, coordinators, and IEC workers. Their tasks might include:

1. Consulting local-level staff to set objectives for each distributor.
2. Establishing and maintaining contact with community leaders.
3. Identifying, selecting and training local-level staff.
4. Providing regular technical assistance to local-level staff in areas such as record-keeping, orientation of users and IEC activities.
5. Visiting distributors regularly to ensure adequate performance in terms of the number of clients and the quality of services offered.
6. Providing contraceptive services, such as insertion of IUDs and injectables, during supervisory visits.
7. Supplying distributors with contraceptives, educational materials and other supplies, as required.
8. Coordinating the activities of the programme with those of other community groups.
9. Holding regular meetings with central-level staff to inform them of programme activities, noting achievements and problems.
10. Monitoring programme activities and analysing the performance of staff in order to identify the actions needed to solve any problems.
11. Documenting the assessments and actions noted for use at supervisory level, for self-evaluation, and for reporting to central-level staff.
12. Providing feedback on performance to distributors.

Community staff

Community staff or distributors are responsible for providing contraceptive services at the community level. Examples of tasks include the following:

1. Participating in the development of individual objectives.

2. Providing information and education to individuals and community groups on the importance of family planning.

3. Helping individuals choose a family planning method appropriate to their needs, preferences, and reproductive and health status.

4. Checking for contraindications to the use of specific methods.

5. Providing clients with more detailed information about their chosen method and with a supply of contraceptives.

6. Referring clients who require clinical services or request other contraceptive methods to appropriate service providers.

7. Maintaining a record of IEC activities, users registered, contraceptives distributed, and referrals made.

Fig. 6. Example of a job description for a CBD distributor

Position (title): CBD distributor.

Primary responsibilities: Providing information about family planning, counselling, and contraceptives to the community.

Specific tasks: (Include all tasks listed in the workplans.) Examples for this position might include:

- Deliver talks on family planning in the community.
- Provide clients with information about specific contraceptive methods and a supply of temporary contraceptives.
- Refer clients requesting other contraceptive methods to clinic-based services.
- Maintain a record of the services delivered to clients, including the number and type of contraceptives distributed.

Qualifications: (These are the minimum qualifications considered necessary to carry out the above tasks.) Examples for this position might include:

- Interested in family planning.
- Resident of the community for at least one year.
- Fluent in the local language.
- Able to work at least 10 hours per week.
- Member of a community organization.
- Currently using a contraceptive method.

Reports to: The assigned supervisor.

Fig. 7. Example of a job description for a CBD supervisor

Position (title): CBD supervisor.

Primary responsibilities: training (initial and refresher), supervising and evaluating the activities of the distributors.

Specific tasks: (Include all tasks listed in the workplans.) Examples for this position might include:

- Identify and recruit distributors.
- Train distributors.
- Set personal goals for distributors.
- Supply distributors with contraceptives and promotional materials, as required.
- Provide technical assistance to distributors.
- Collect service data and prepare monthly reports.
- Conduct IEC sessions in the community.
- Conduct refresher training.

Qualifications: (These are the minimum qualifications considered necessary to carry out the above tasks.) Examples for this position might include:

- At least one year's experience in health or family planning service delivery.
- Fluent in the local language.
- Able to read and write.
- Interested in family planning.
- Currently using a contraceptive method.
- Previous work in community development.

Reports to: The programme manager.

8. Collaborating with intermediate-level staff in coordinating the activities of the programme with those of other community groups.

9. Following up individuals who drop out of the programme or who do not follow through with a referral.

After performing task analysis, the programme manager can develop job descriptions for each position and proceed to select personnel. Figs. 6 and 7 are examples of job descriptions for a CBD distributor and supervisor, which may be adapted according to the needs of the programme.

Selecting and training personnel

Selection

Selecting field personnel for community-based programmes places unusual demands on the programme manager. While most staffing requirements at the central level are routine, selection criteria change considerably at the supervisory and community levels. This is because staff at these levels must have certain qualities that are often hard to identify without extensive interviews and references (see Fig. 8).

In many CBD programmes, programme managers have found that while the organization's existing procedures are usually adequate for selecting central and intermediate staff, a different approach is needed for selecting local staff.

Individuals selected to work at the local level must be acceptable to community leaders and to the target group within the community. This may mean that they must have a particular ethnic or tribal affiliation, be well known in the community, be trusted by others as a reliable source of information, be able to speak a certain language, or live in a particular location, etc. Thus, it is important that programme managers seek assistance from community leaders in the selection process.

Many successful CBD programmes select local-level staff by asking recognized community leaders, such as mayors and village chiefs, to recommend appropriate people and by approaching influential community members, such as teachers, traditional birth attendants, shopkeepers and political leaders, to be CBD promoters. It is important that both the community and the organization are satisfied that the local-level staff can

Fig. 8. Qualities of successful field staff

Distributor
- Practises family planning.
- Respected member of the community.
- A peer of the clients.
- Accepted by local leaders.

Supervisor
- Understands local culture and language.
- Accepted by local leaders.
- Previous experience as a distributor.
- Good communication skills (writing, speaking).

provide high-quality services according to the community's needs.

In addition, programme managers will need to determine the amount of time the prospective local staff have available, whether they are willing to work as volunteers and whether they are able to meet the needs and requirements of the programme.

Training

All staff involved in the CBD programme will require some kind of training. For example, distributors will need training in how to procure and distribute contraceptives in the community; statisticians will need instruction in the objectives of the CBD programme and how to monitor and evaluate the programme; and clinic personnel will need training in how to process and document referrals from distributors. To determine the training requirements for staff at each level, the programme manager should consult the job descriptions, which list the specific tasks for which the various staff members are responsible. The training they receive should be based on these tasks. While staff members need general information about family planning and about the CBD programme, their training should focus on the tasks they are expected to perform. This approach is called competency-based training.

The training of central-level staff of the programme is usually similar to that of other health-delivery programmes. However, there are a number of significant differences at the supervisory and community levels, where the emphasis is on training through practical experience and independent problem-solving. There are several reasons for this:

1. Because the programme is based in the community, the quality must be highest at that level.

2. Distributors are usually volunteers who have little or no previous formal training, and are often illiterate.

3. Supervisors and distributors must be able to make decisions on their own, since they will not usually be able to consult senior staff.

Therefore, supervisors and distributors must be capable of carrying out their routine tasks and coping with unexpected situations without continual assistance from others. Because of the interpersonal nature of CBD work, role-playing exercises are used extensively in their training. In this way, these staff become accustomed to solving problems by themselves, and become confident in their ability to make decisions on their own.

Most importantly, both supervisors and distributors are responsible for many different tasks and should not be burdened with information they will not use. Their training should prepare them for specific tasks according to established protocols, and to achieve the performance standards required by the programme.

Although many different approaches to training CBD workers have been developed, most programmes have recognized that a two-stage approach is most effective, consisting of initial training and periodic refresher training.

Initial training

Initial training for supervisors and distributors is conducted over a specified period, covering the basic elements listed in Figs. 9 and 10.

Training will differ, depending upon whether the individuals involved are literate or not, whether they are voluntary or paid, and whether they have prior experience in family planning or health. In some cases, one day may be the most that a housewife or barber can spare for training, while in others, paid CBD workers may be able to spend several weeks acquiring skills.

Initial training may be conducted by outside consultants specialized in training non-professional community health workers. This approach is often used for the information and

Fig. 9. Basic elements of training for CBD distributors

- Goals and objectives of the institution.
- Health and economic benefits of birth spacing.
- Characteristics of available contraceptive methods.
- Screening for contraindications (see page 58).
- Referral procedures, and sources of referral-related services.
- Record-keeping (and simple accounting procedures, if fees are collected).
- Counselling skills and techniques to encourage family planning.
- Skills for promoting the programme in the community.
- Basic reproductive anatomy and physiology.

Fig. 10. Basic elements of training for CBD supervisors

All of the elements listed in Fig. 9, with the following additional subjects:

- Supervision (see page 53).
- Techniques for motivating volunteer distributors (see page 54).
- Techniques for developing support from the community.
- Reporting procedures and forms.
- Training skills.

Fig. 11. Traditional birth attendants receiving training from a nurse

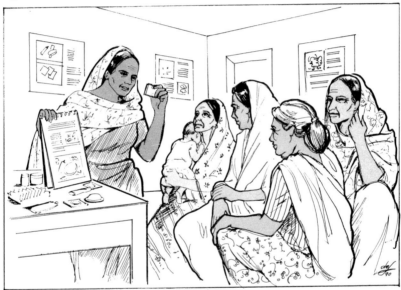

educational components of training. However, in most cases, experienced distributors, supervisors and programme coordinators train new staff.

The formal training often takes place over a very short period of time (1–3 days), during which the essential elements of contraceptive distribution are covered (Fig. 11). For example, in the CBD programmes operated by Family of the Future in Egypt and PROFAMILIA in Colombia, the formal training for distributors lasts one day and covers only the essential elements of distribution. In contrast, in the CBD programme that is run by the Zimbabwe National Family Planning Council, the formal training for distributors lasts 4 weeks.

After the formal training, the trainees receive in-service instruction: new supervisors accompany experienced supervisors on their rounds; new distributors observe experienced distributors at work and receive instruction from supervisors.

Refresher training

Some programmes try to teach too much in the initial training sessions, and overlook the importance of follow-up training. This includes refresher training on topics covered during the initial training session, and training on new topics as the needs of distributors and the programme change. Often this is provided by the supervisor as a component of individual or group supervision.

In many programmes, supervisory staff arrange one-day meetings with groups of experienced distributors in order to answer their questions and to share their experiences.

Regardless of the approach chosen, the basic elements of initial and refresher training are the same (see Fig. 12).

Fig. 12. Basic elements of initial and refresher training for CBD staff

1. Analyse the tasks involved and the performance standards required (see page 43).

2. Design and implement a training programme:

   - Decide the content of the training programme.
   - Prepare the learning objectives.
   - Select the teaching methods to be used.
   - Develop the curriculum.
   - Develop the teaching materials.
   - Conduct the training programme.
   - Assess the trainees.

3. Evaluate the programme:

   - Conduct periodic follow-up visits to CBD workers to assess their performance and knowledge.
   - Modify the initial training programme as needed.
   - Provide refresher and in-service training to reinforce basic skills and teach new ones.

Source: Adapted from Terborgh et al. (1990) *A model of training and quality control in community-based family planning programs.*

Supervision

Supervision is essential for maintaining both the quality of the programme and motivation among staff. To be successful, supervision should be helpful and positive rather than punitive and controlling. To ensure that staff are aware of their supervisory responsibilities as well as who their supervisor is, programme managers should include this information in the job description.

If the supervisor is a trained health professional, he or she may provide clinical services such as IUD insertion or injectable contraception during supervisory visits to the distributors. The services can then be scheduled to coincide with these visits.

Scheduling supervisory visits

There is no universally accepted rule governing the frequency and length of supervisory visits; indeed, it has been found that the quality of the visits is more important than the quantity. In one CBD programme, it was found that the ratio of distributors to supervisors had no significant effect on the performance of the distributors. However, the same study reported that increased supervision had a positive influence on all CBD services except referrals.

Another programme found that increased supervision had a negative effect on service performance. The most effective approach appears to be periodic supervisory visits lasting 1–2 days, combined with meetings among groups of distributors.

CBD programmes generally establish a schedule for supervisory visits, since distributors usually work part-time. However, unscheduled visits are also made occasionally. Supervisors should be available to local staff, as needed, for technical assistance. Ideally, the supervisor should observe the distributor at work, although this may require staying in the village for a day or more.

It is essential that supervisors spend most of their time visiting distributors. Therefore, the reporting requirements should not impose unreasonable burdens on supervisors and should respect their limited time and busy schedules.

Knowing the community

Supervisors should be familiar with the communities the programme serves and actively assist the distributors in developing

53

and maintaining community support. The supervisor should therefore understand how the communities function and establish contact with influential community leaders and groups to gain their support for the programme.

Personal planning conference

The concept of the "personal planning conference" (PPC) provides supervisors with a useful tool for supervision. It is based on the assumption that people are more motivated to accomplish goals set by themselves rather than goals set by others. In periodic PPCs, supervisors collaborate with their distributors to develop personal service-delivery goals based on the objectives of the organization. The PPC also provides a forum for supervisors and distributors to solve any problems together.

Guidelines for conducting a PPC are given in Fig. 13, while Fig. 14 provides a model checklist for conducting a PPC.

Motivating volunteer workers

One of the biggest challenges facing CBD programme managers is how to maintain motivation among volunteer distribu-

Fig. 13. Guidelines for conducting a personal planning conference

- It is the distributor's time. Listen to his or her opinions. Ask what helped and hindered progress.
- Keep the discussion focused on future activities. Discuss how improvements might be made, and what the distributor feels would help.
- When it is your turn to talk, be open and honest.
- Agree on the goals to be achieved during the next period and how to measure them.
- Ensure that the goals are feasible and achievable to avoid discouraging the distributor. Remember, setting goals means making a commitment to change. This may concern some distributors.
- Find out exactly how the distributor intends to reach each goal and what actions are planned.
- Share ideas with the distributor on how best to reach the goals and suggest various approaches.
- Finally, review and put in writing the goals and measurements agreed upon, and the timing of your next visit. Give a copy to the distributor.

Fig. 14. Checklist for conducting a personal planning conference

---

Personal planning conference checklist

Distributor _____   Date _____
District _____   Village _____

1. Review activities

Review the previous PPC checklist with the distributor, including his or her personal targets and any follow-up issues that were to be addressed between supervisory visits.

Review the service data:

- Is the distributor recording data properly?
- How is the distributor performing in relation to his or her personal targets?
- What IEC and promotional activities have been conducted?
- Are there sufficient contraceptives and are they being stored properly?

2. Evaluate performance

- Will the personal targets be missed, met or exceeded?
- What factors have enhanced performance?
- What factors have adversely affected performance?
- Have there been any changes in the community that might have affected service delivery (e.g. new service providers; resistance to CBD or family planning; social, economic or health-related factors)?

3. Plan for the future

- On the basis of the review and the evaluation, are any changes needed (e.g. in user targets, IEC strategy, contraceptives offered, etc.)?
- What kinds of support would help the distributor perform better (e.g. more frequent resupply of contraceptives; assistance in outreach activities; better access to transport, IEC materials or medical back-up)?

4. List revised personal targets: _____

5. Assign issues for follow-up:

Supervisor: _____
Distributor: _____

tors. Programmes with high drop-out rates among their distributors must face the expense of continually recruiting and training new staff. Furthermore, unhappy distributors do not perform well and have difficulty generating interest in family planning.

The following are proven incentives that, when managed carefully, can make the programme a success.

1. Most people will volunteer to join what they perceive to be an important effort. Volunteer distributors must feel that they are needed, and are making an important contribution to the programme's success. Therefore, it is essential that they receive adequate support and positive feedback from supervisors.

2. Similarly, volunteer distributors enjoy the prestige of their association with the organization. Make the most of this by providing them with items bearing the logo of the organization, such as signs advertising their services, laboratory coats or cases.

3. Encouraging team spirit has proven extremely successful in many programmes. Friendly competitions are held among distributors and awards ceremonies are staged, during which recognition is given to as many distributors and supervisors as time permits.

4. Make the distributors' job as easy as possible by providing adequate support. They must be helped to develop a strong foundation of community support, and backed by an effective promotional campaign to generate demand for their services. Technical support and a source of medical back-up should be available. It is also essential that the distributors be resupplied regularly with contraceptives and educational materials.

5. Most CBD programmes now charge fees for their contraceptives, and allow distributors to keep a fixed percentage (commonly 50%) of the receipts as an incentive. In general, such payments are not large enough to motivate many distributors, although they may be sufficiently large to do so for those at the lowest economic level. However, profit-sharing schemes are usually less effective at motivating distributors than the other approaches described here.

Providing feedback

It is essential that distributors receive regular feedback from their supervisors regarding their work and what is expected of them. Similarly, supervisory staff should receive regular feedback from central-level staff.

Counselling

The quality of counselling is crucial, and can determine whether the programme will fail or succeed. Its purpose is to assist the client to make an informed, voluntary, well-considered decision regarding family planning. During counselling, the distributor provides clients with information about family planning and other important health-related issues, such as the acquired immunodeficiency syndrome (AIDS) and oral rehydration therapy. Such information should be accurate and should be presented in an effective and sympathetic manner. This is especially important in remote areas, since the distributor may be the only source of information for clients.

Through counselling, the distributor:

- Provides clients with information about family planning, responsible parenthood, and the health, social and economic benefits of birth spacing.
- Provides information about available methods of contraception, their comparative advantages and disadvantages, and their possible side-effects.
- Recommends appropriate methods for the clients to choose.
- Provides information about techniques to prevent the transmission of HIV and other sexually transmitted diseases.
- Provides guidance to users who have questions or complaints, request a change in method, or are suffering from contraceptive-related side-effects.
- Arranges referrals for other contraceptive methods and clinical services.

One of the most important aspects of CBD counselling is the interview with clients requesting oral contraceptives.

First, it is essential that women who wish to use the pill are carefully screened for contraindications and, if necessary, provided with a choice of suitable alternative methods.

Secondly, precisely because of the importance of the screening procedure, this is the primary front upon which CBD programmes receive criticism from the medical community. To ensure that the interview is conducted properly, most programmes provide distributors with some form of checklist as a guide.

Designing the checklist provides an opportunity to involve the medical community and medical staff from the CBD organization. An example of such a checklist, adapted from one designed by the Kenya Family Planning Private Sector Programme, is given in Fig. 15.

Fig. 15. Checklist for screening clients for contraindications to the use of oral contraceptives

---

This checklist must be completed for any new female client who wishes to use oral contraceptives (the pill). If the answer to ALL of the questions below is "No", you may give her the pill. If the answer to ANY question is "Yes", you MUST refer her to a doctor or nurse for an examination before she can be given the pill. In the meantime she must be provided with an alternative form of contraception, such as condoms or spermicidal foam. Save the completed checklist as your permanent record of this interview.

You do NOT have to complete this checklist for continuing pill users, but you should always ask continuing users if they have had any problems before resupplying them.

Questions	Yes	No
Are you over 40 years of age?	—	—
Are you a heavy smoker (over 20 cigarettes a day)?	—	—
Are you breast-feeding a baby?	—	—
Do you ever have seizures (fits)?	—	—
Do you ever have pain in your legs?	—	—
Do you ever have swollen legs (oedema)?	—	—
Do you have visible (varicose) veins in your legs?	—	—
Do you ever suffer from chest pains?	—	—
Are you very short of breath after hard work or strenuous exercise?	—	—
Do you suffer from bad headaches?	—	—
Have you ever been told by a health worker not to use the pill?	—	—
Have you ever had a blood clot, a heart attack, or a stroke?	—	—
Is your skin or are your eyes abnormally yellow?	—	—
Do you have a history of high blood pressure?	—	—

If the answer to any of these questions is YES, you should see a doctor or nurse before using the pill. This does NOT mean anything is wrong with you, only that the pill may not be the best choice for you.

Name and address of client:

Source: Adapted from Kenya Family Planning Private Sector Programme. Used by permission.

Making referrals

CBD programmes have direct access to communities, which enables them to identify people in need of services who would have been reached only with great difficulty by clinic-based programmes. Therefore, distributors must be trained to recognize clients in need of higher level services and to make referrals to the appropriate service provider.

A good referral system depends on three essential elements:

- Well-trained distributors who identify clients in need of additional services, and then refer them to the most appropriate source of those services.
- The availability of well equipped facilities and the cooperation of staff at the referral site.
- An effective system of follow-up to ensure that clients attend for services.

Learning Point

APROSAMI, the national family planning organization of Peru, found that clinical services expanded because of the large number of referrals, particularly for IUDs, generated by its distributors. Although the distributors are volunteers, they receive economic incentives based on the number of referrals made for clinical services (IUDs and voluntary sterilization), as well as a percentage of contraceptive sales.

Follow-up

Follow-up ensures that clients who have been referred for clinical services attend the service facility, and receive the desired service and any additional care that may be needed.

Most programmes use a referral card system of follow-up. An example of such a card system is shown in Fig. 16.

A typical follow-up system works in the following way:

1. The card is completed by the distributor, who gives the clients their copy and directs them to the source of services.

2. Upon arrival at the clinical facility, the clients present their copy of the referral card at the reception (Fig. 17).

3. After the clients receive the requested services, their cards are filed by the clinic.

59

Fig. 16. An example of a referral card system

Referral card	Referral card
Name of client:	Name of client:
Address:	Address:
Reason for referral:	Reason for referral:
Name and address of service facility:	Name and address of service facility:
Name and address of distributor:	Name and address of distributor:
Date: Time:	Date: Time:
Distributor's copy	Client's copy

4. The distributors, in turn, give their copy of the referral cards to the supervisor when they present their monthly log-book. Many programmes reward distributors for completed referrals with small payments or other incentives.

5. The supervisor then checks with the clinical facility to determine which clients did not appear for services at the appointed time.

6. The supervisor notifies the distributor responsible who, in turn, conducts a follow-up visit (or other form of contact) to those clients. Depending upon the situation, the distributor may provide more counselling, and then reschedule or cancel the referral.

Follow-up is also conducted to find out why clients have stopped visiting the distributor for resupply. Clients may drop out of CBD programmes for various reasons, such as moving to a new community, disapproval of the spouse or family, desire to have another child, shyness, living far from the distribution point, and contraceptive-related side-effects.

Fig. 17. Clients presenting their referral cards at the clinic

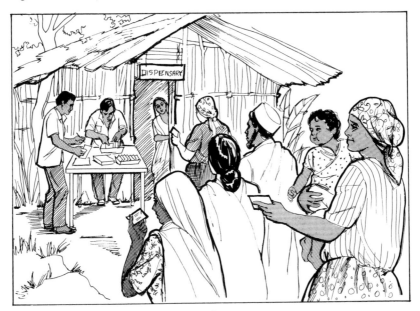

By following up such clients, the distributor or supervisor can find ways to improve service delivery, and can provide valuable support to users who may be shy about continuing with family planning, need to change methods, or who are simply misinformed about the risks of oral contraceptives.

However, the nature and extent of follow-up depends on the local setting and culture. Whereas some programmes follow up all clients who drop out or who do not attend for services, others feel that follow-up is a waste of staff time or intrudes upon the privacy of clients.

Information, education and communication activities

Informing the community about family planning and about the availability of services will encourage more people to use family planning methods. Many CBD programmes have found that the two most successful information channels are local staff and satisfied clients (word of mouth).

While these channels are important, programmes can benefit substantially, especially when they are just starting, from a carefully targeted IEC campaign that can "spread the word" rapidly and in a culturally acceptable manner.

Target groups

To be most effective, IEC activities must be focused on groups in which the prevalence of contraceptive use is low. Possible target groups include students, new mothers, women who are breast-feeding, young married couples, men, or people considered to be at risk of HIV infection and other sexually transmitted diseases.

Information channels

To identify effective channels through which to convey information about family planning, the programme manager should find out how information is conveyed, both formally and informally, within the community or target group.

Among the information channels that have been used successfully by CBD programmes are community organizations, mothers' clubs, sports clubs, associations, schools, markets, traditional healers, women's and men's hairdressers, social events, and community meetings.

In addition to the information channels listed above, which rely on interpersonal communication, there are usually a variety of media channels through which family planning and the CBD programme may be promoted. Table 3 lists these channels, together with their respective advantages and disadvantages. The choice of medium should be based on the local environment, the target groups, the nature of the message, and the relative cost.

Many communities provide support in the form of free radio and television time, newspaper space, printing and design work. Furthermore, family planning organizations can receive free publicity by sending well written press releases to newspapers, magazines and radio stations, or by staging events that attract the attention of the media.

In planning an IEC strategy, programme managers should consider the following questions.

- Where and how do members of the target community receive information (e.g. from newspapers, radio, health professionals, neighbours, leaflets distributed at the market, or community meetings)?

Table 3. Advantages and disadvantages of selected media for promoting family planning

Medium	Advantages	Disadvantages
Radio	Effective means of reaching the public, even in remote areas; lends prestige; and free air time often available. News and talk shows often looking for topical stories.	Air time and production of recurrent radio spots can be costly. Message hard to tailor to specific groups because of the diversity of the audience.
Television	Similar to radio, but allows a visual element to be incorporated.	Similar to radio, but much more costly. Usually provides only limited access to low-income groups.
Newspapers and magazines	Popular sources of information for all income groups. Public health messages are often printed free of charge, particularly if sent in the form of a press release.	Directly reach only literate persons; messages usually put in obscure page location and appear for only one day.
Leaflets, posters and billboards	Most popular and inexpensive media for promoting CBD; messages can be designed for specific groups and distributed in target areas. Very effective way to inform public of service locations and opening hours.	May be expensive to produce in large quantities. Must be pretested to ensure effectiveness and acceptability.
Promotional gifts, e.g. key-rings, pens, T-shirts, calendars, with printed messages	If well designed, such items can be very popular and often continue to be used for many years, thus providing prolonged exposure for the message.	Costly to design and produce in large quantities. Usually only very simple messages can be delivered.

- What information do people need about family planning (e.g. its importance for maternal health and child survival, its economic benefits to the family, or the advantages and disadvantages of available contraceptive methods)?

- What do they need to know about the CBD programme (e.g. what methods are offered, or the location of the community distribution posts)?

- Who needs this information (e.g. community leaders, potential clients, couples, or single men and women)?

- Which information channels would be most effective for providing this information?

- What are people expected to do with this information (e.g. decide to plan their families, use CBD services, encourage others to use family planning, or try new methods of contraception)?

These questions can best be answered by interviewing key members of the community, by reviewing the experiences of other health programmes, and by assessing the resources available.

One of the most effective ways to answer these questions is through the use of focus groups. Focus groups are in-depth discussions involving 6–10 people from the target audience with similar backgrounds or interests. Under the guidance of a moderator, topics related to family planning are discussed. The objective is to learn what people want to know, how this information can best be presented to them, and how they will use the information.

Focus group discussions are conducted as open-ended sessions, usually 1–2 hours in length, in which participants are encouraged to comment on the topics, to ask questions, and to respond to others' comments. The sessions enable programme staff to hear and observe the groups' reactions to the topics and to gain insight into the participants' knowledge, beliefs, and concepts. Focus groups are particularly useful in CBD with its emphasis on community involvement, in that the community develops its own messages and identifies the best ways for communicating them.

There are numerous publications on designing, testing, implementing and evaluating information, education and communication activities. In addition, several specialized organizations provide technical assistance in this area. The addresses of these agencies are listed in Annex 7.

Establishing a logistics system

Since the purpose of CBD is to extend contraceptive services to areas with limited access to family planning services, continuity of supplies is essential. A well managed logistics system is especially important in the context of CBD in that the supply chain can become extended and extra attention must be given to monitoring the expiry dates of the contraceptives. It is also essential to monitor supplies because of the informal nature of contraceptive distribution by non-professionals.

In many cases, when a new CBD programme is started, organizations that already have a logistics system in place may decide to use that system for the new products as well. If this approach is chosen, there are some issues that are unique to family planning commodities and to CBD that must be considered.

This section discusses four aspects of logistics that will ensure that the CBD programme runs smoothly and offers a dependable supply of contraceptives to its clients: calculating contraceptive requirements; procurement; storing supplies; and establishing an inventory system.

Calculating contraceptive requirements

Forecasting contraceptive requirements, particularly for a new or very large programme, can be a difficult and time-consuming exercise. However, with some care and practice, programme managers can become reasonably proficient at calculating the kinds and amounts of contraceptives needed by the programme.

The exercise should be performed immediately upon setting the objectives of the programme. There are two steps in determining contraceptive requirements: (i) determining the mix of methods; and (ii) estimating the potential demand for each method.

Determining the mix of methods. Community-based programmes offer only a limited variety of contraceptive methods appropriate for distribution by non-professionals, usually oral contraceptives, condoms, and other barrier contraceptives such as spermicidal foams, jellies, tablets and suppositories. Distributors may also provide information about natural methods of family planning. However, the popularity of each method can vary enormously between regions, countries, and even communities.

To determine which are the most popular contraceptives in a community, programme managers may use one or several of the following methods:

- Review service records of the existing family planning programme.

- Talk to local pharmacists or chemists.

- Look at the age structure of the population.

- Conduct a small survey in the community.

- Experiment through a small-scale programme.

Typically, a CBD programme might offer the following mix of contraceptive methods:

—40% oral contraceptives (80% low-dose; 20% standard dosage);

—30% condoms (often varies widely, depending on locality);[1]

—20% other barrier methods (e.g. foaming tablets, foams, jellies and suppositories);

—10% referrals for other methods.

Estimating the potential demand for each method. Table 4 indicates the estimated annual contraceptive requirements per user, by method.

Table 4. Estimated annual contraceptive requirements per user, by method

Method	Estimated annual requirements per user
Oral contraceptives	13 cycles
Condoms	144 pieces
Foaming tablets	144 tablets
Foams, creams, jellies	6 tubes (25 applications per tube)

---

[1] Given the growing demand for condoms for the prevention of sexually transmitted diseases, including HIV infection, this figure may be substantially higher.

Procurement

Procurement of the necessary commodities might be a simple matter if the organization is already providing family planning services to the community. However, if family planning services are new to the organization, it may be more difficult to obtain adequate supplies. Fig. 18 provides a checklist for procuring contraceptive supplies. In general, sources of supply consist of:

- Purchases from local pharmaceutical firms.

Fig. 18. Checklist for procuring contraceptives

1. Determine the brands of modern, approved contraceptives most popular in the country.

2. Determine if the brands are available locally. Talk to representatives from local pharmaceutical firms. They may be willing to provide the contraceptives at very low cost, on the basis that it is better to help promote wider acceptance of their products than to risk increased competition from other brands. Try to obtain fixed-price guarantees for as long as possible.

3. If not available locally, determine if the product, or a similar one, is available from international donor agencies. The addresses of these agencies are listed in Annex 5. Remember, it can take many months for orders to arrive, even from local firms. Therefore the initial supplies should be ordered as soon as the service objectives have been set and the projected mix of methods determined.

4. Identify a reliable source of supply of contraceptives and maintain good communications with the sales representative.

5. Agree on the timing of regular orders, and procedures for making emergency orders.

6. Make sure that the storage facility is ready and that it conforms to accepted standards for storing contraceptives.

7. If the contraceptives are to be imported, enquire about which ports are the easiest to import through (i.e. where delays due to customs requirements etc. are kept to a minimum).

8. Find out exactly how the products must be described on the bill of lading to satisfy customs requirements. If the crates are labelled differently from the customs documents provided, the shipments may be returned or delayed.

9. If necessary, make arrangements for a customs-clearing agency to help clear the shipment. However, determine beforehand whether the donor or the organization will pay for this service.

10. Determine in advance how the goods will be transported from the port to the storage facility. Remember that most donors will not pay for inland freight.

- Purchases from international manufacturers.

- Contributions from international agencies (see Annex 5).

Each source has certain advantages and disadvantages. However, the two most important factors in deciding which source to use are the quality of the product and the preferences of the clients. Many CBD programmes have performed poorly because of low acceptance of the products that were offered.

For example, for several years the family planning organization CEMOPLAF of Ecuador was unsuccessful in promoting its CBD services. Few users were recruited and those that were usually dropped out. Many potential users were found to be requesting a local brand of oral contraceptive. Finally, the programme manager decided to offer the local brand instead of a donated brand. The local brand was purchased from a local pharmaceutical firm. The result was an immediate growth in the CBD programme, and the organization developed a self-sustaining revolving fund that uses income from fees for purchasing the contraceptives.

Similarly, in Bangladesh, private CBD programmes increased the prevalence of contraceptive use by offering locally procured low-dose pills that were unavailable from government health posts.

Goods procured abroad are by nature subject to unpredictable problems such as bureaucratic and processing delays, customs duties, and inland freight. Frequently, commodities are damaged or pilfered in customs warehouses, and may be exposed to heat, rain and other elements.

Requesting commodities from international agencies. A list of international agencies that donate contraceptives is provided in Annex 5. Programme managers should write to the agencies directly to request assistance and a copy of the agency's request form. Most agencies have request forms in which the programme manager provides information about the CBD programme, including its size and its contraceptive requirements, and details about procedures for shipping to the particular country. (For detailed information about procuring condoms, see WHO, 1994a.)

Once the request form has been completed, it should be returned to the agency for review and approval. In some instances, the agency will be unable to supply specific kinds and brands of requested commodities. For example, a locally popular oral contraceptive may be requested that is manufactured locally, or that is not stocked by the donor. In this case, the request must either be modified in accordance with the agency's recommendations, or sent elsewhere.

Programme managers should inform the agency of any customs regulations and unusual circumstances that affect shipments to the country. Examples include specific ports of entry that seem to clear shipments quickly; special circumstances that would indicate a preference for shipment by air rather than sea; or labelling recommendations. In one country, a shipment of plastic IUDs was refused entry because of a ban on imports of any petroleum-based (including plastic) manufactured products.

Once the request has been approved, the commodities will be sent by air or ocean freight. The type of transport employed usually depends on the size and weight of the order or on other factors, such as the shorter customs clearance procedures at certain ports of entry, time considerations, or accessibility of inland transport.

The recipient organization will be notified by the supplier of the mode of transportation, the name of the carrier, the approximate date of arrival, and the port at which the commodities will arrive.

As the consignee of the shipment, the recipient organization will be sent the shipping documents that are necessary for clearing customs. If another agency will be receiving the commodities on behalf of the recipient organization, that agency becomes the consignee and will be sent the shipping documents.

For shipments by sea, the recipient organization (or other designated consignee) will be sent a *bill of lading*. For shipments by air, an *air waybill* will be sent. A "letter of contribution" (also known as a "gift certification") may also be required, stating that the shipment is a donation and therefore not subject to import duties and restrictions.

Storing supplies

Contraceptives are valuable and vital to the success of the programme. Care must therefore be taken to store and account for them properly.

Supplies should be stored in a well ventilated, dry, clean area. The temperature should not exceed 24 °C, and the supplies should be protected from sunlight. Shipping containers should be stored 10 cm above ground level, preferably on pallets, and

Fig. 19. Storing contraceptive supplies

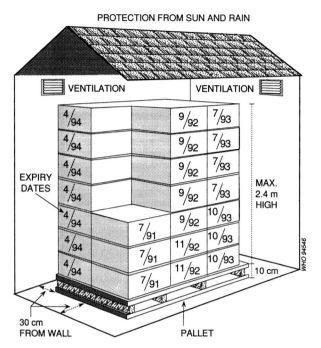

PROTECTION FROM SUN AND RAIN

should not be stacked higher than 2.4 m. They should be away from the walls. The containers should be clearly labelled and the expiry dates of the products should be visible (see Fig. 19). As a general rule, the older supplies should be issued before the newer supplies (the "first in–first out" system) to prevent spoilage. To ensure that this is done properly, new contraceptives should be placed behind the older commodities in the storeroom. (For detailed information about storing condoms, see United States: Department of Health and Human Services, 1993 and WHO, 1994b.)

Establishing an inventory system

An inventory system is essential to allow the programme manager to monitor stock levels at each level of the programme. Fig. 20 provides an example of a simple current inventory system designed to enable distributors to know at a glance what stock they have available, what they have received and distributed, and when they will need to order more supplies.

70

Fig. 20. A sample inventory report form

Distributor:	Personal identification no.:

Inventory report for the month:

A	B	C	D	E	F	G
Product	Amount available at start of month	Amount issued	New stock level (B − C)	Amount added	Amount available at end of month (D + E)	Amount ordered

If an existing inventory system is used, there are several points that programme managers should consider:

- Keep family planning commodities separate from other supplies.

- Train the supply staff to recognize the different products, expiry dates, package sizes, and routing information.

- Incinerate or bury any contraceptives that have passed their expiry date.

- Train supply and supervisory staff about recommended re-stocking levels for distributors, and the importance of making periodic checks of distributors' stocks to ensure that supply reflects demand, and that expiry dates are not exceeded.

5. Monitoring and evaluating the programme

This chapter explains how to establish a data collection system for monitoring and evaluating the performance of the programme in terms of the service-delivery output and the consumption of resources. Examples of indicators for monitoring and evaluating the programme are provided, together with sources of data. An indicator that is becoming increasingly popular is the "couple–years of protection" (CYP); and the chapter provides simple instructions for assessing service-delivery data in terms of the CYP.

Monitoring is the term used for the continuous follow-up of activities to ensure that they are proceeding according to plan. Information gained from monitoring is used for evaluation. Evaluation is the systematic assessment of the relevance, progress, effectiveness, and impact of a particular course of action. Effective systems for monitoring and evaluation are essential to ensure that services are proceeding as planned. Through the process of evaluation, the programme manager learns what progress has been made towards the objectives of the programme, what factors aided or impeded progress, how effective the programmed activities were in terms of expenditure of resources, and how to improve the quality of performance in the future.

Both monitoring and evaluation depend, for the most part, on similar indicators and sources of data. However, since evaluations are conducted to determine the impact of the programme in relation to its objectives, they often require additional information that is generated outside the programme, e.g. a community survey that measures changes in the prevalence of contraceptive use.

Monitoring the programme

Monitoring and evaluation are based on service data. This section discusses the kinds of data needed for monitoring the programme, and some of the ways in which data are analysed and used at each level of the programme.

Analysis of service data allows the programme manager to monitor the performance of the programme in relation to its objectives. It also permits the manager to see the effects of alternative service strategies and to allocate programme resources accordingly to maximize performance.

However, service data must be recorded accurately and reported promptly to be useful. Frequently, problems arise because the field staff who are responsible for recording the data have a poor understanding of the importance accorded the data by the central office.

All staff must understand why they are collecting data, how the data are used to provide information about the programme, who will use the information, and how the information will help them succeed at their own job. Therefore, it is essential that all staff involved in recording or analysing service data thoroughly understand both the programme's service objectives and the reporting requirements.

After the service data have been returned to the central office, they are analysed and used to evaluate the performance of the programme in relation to its objectives. Reports, both internal and external, are prepared as necessary. The results are then communicated back through the various levels of the programme, including coordinators, supervisors and distributors.

Programme managers must look at a variety of measures, both quantitative and qualitative, to make informed decisions about the programme. Therefore, they should ensure that the needed data are recorded. This means that the data recording forms used by the programme staff must be designed accordingly.

The various programme elements for which measurements are needed are discussed below.

Service delivery

Numerical data related to service objectives provide the manager with the basic indicators for monitoring the programme. Examples of service-delivery measures include the number of users registered, the quantity and types of contraceptives distributed, and the number of referrals made. One such measure that is being increasingly widely used is the "couple–years of protection" (CYP). (For further discussion of this measure, see page 79).

Another critical measure is programme coverage in terms of the change, over time, in contraceptive use in the community served by the CBD programme. This measure must be anticipated from the start of the programme, either by noting the prevalence rate found in the community during a recent survey, or by conducting a small-scale survey of knowledge, awareness and practice of contraception among the local population. (See Annex 3 for a model of a simple survey.)

Service quality

Data on the quality of the services provided are also important for monitoring purposes. Examples of service-quality measures include growth in the number of continuing users and a reduction in the drop-out rate among distributors. However, the easiest way for programme managers to measure quality is to monitor the number of users who list "heard from a satisfied client" when asked how they became aware of the programme. If clients are literate, programme managers may also use anonymous multiple-choice questionnaires to determine whether there have been any unplanned pregnancies among clients, and whether they are satisfied with the location of the distribution points, the methods offered, etc.

Use of resources

Cost. Cost is an important measure that is frequently overlooked. By comparing the costs involved in providing services through alternative service-delivery strategies, the programme manager can improve the allocation of resources. The simplest and most practical measure of cost is the total recurrent (operating) costs per user or per couple–years of protection attributable to the programme.

Staff time. Measurements of time worked can provide the programme manager with important information about the efficiency with which services are provided. Examples of such measures include the amount of time spent by distributors per user served, travel time involved in supervisory visits, or the time required to prepare reports. Many programmes require that paid staff keep a record of their time spent per activity, and some ask their distributors to account for their time as well.

Other factors that affect performance

Programme managers must also monitor any other factors that might affect the ability of the programme to achieve its objectives. Examples might include changes in the community or in the availability of resources.

Example

The exercise below is intended to illustrate how a programme is monitored in practice. The first step is to determine what measurements are *essential* for monitoring progress towards an objective, what measurements are *useful* for monitoring the programme, and what measurements are *not necessary* (see Table 5).

Objective: "To register 12 000 new family planning users and provide 8360 couple–years of protection (CYP) through 180 existing CBD posts, 60 new posts, and a new strategy of home visits."
The measurements that are needed for monitoring progress towards this objective are:

—the number of new users registered;
—the number of couple–years of protection provided;
—the number of new CBD posts established;
—the total number of CBD posts.

Assume that the data collected within the first 3 months of implementing the programme show that:

—3421 new users were registered;
—1102 couple–years of protection have been provided;
—39 new CBD distributors have been recruited and trained;
—30 existing CBD distributors have dropped out of the programme.

Analysis of these data indicates that the programme is performing well in some areas and is encountering problems in other areas: the number of new users registered and the number of new distributors recruited are greater than anticipated, while the number of contraceptives distributed is lower than predicted, and there is a high rate of drop-out among distributors.

Table 5. Indicators of programme performance

Measurements	Source of data
Measurements *essential* for monitoring progress towards objectives	
The number of new users registered.	Supervisors' monthly service reports.
The number of couple–years of protection provided.	
The number of new CBD posts established, and the total number of CBD posts.	
Measurements *useful* for monitoring the programme	
The number of users served in each service area (to compare results of alternative service-delivery strategies).	Reports of area or regional meetings of supervisors.
The amount of time spent by field staff per user served (to measure changes in efficiency).	Time sheets for supervisors and distributors; supervisors' monthly service reports.
Cost per couple–year of protection (to monitor changes in cost–effectiveness).	Total recurrent (operating) costs, from quarterly and annual financial reports; distributors' reports; inventory records.
The percentage of users that heard about the programme through the IEC campaign (to measure the effectiveness of the campaign).	Client questionnaires, and small-scale surveys.
Measurements *not necessary* for monitoring the programme	
Marital status of user; age of spouse.	(This kind of information is often collected needlessly, diverting staff from more important activities, such as supervision and service.)

The next step is to determine how to record, collect and analyse the data needed to monitor the programme. The questions that must be answered are:

- Who is responsible for recording, collecting and analysing the data?
- When and where are the data recorded, collected and analysed?
- Who receives the resulting information?
- How is that information used?

Table 6 indicates how information is used at each level of the programme.

Central-level staff

The director uses information to monitor the validity of the programme in relation to the needs of the community, and to determine whether the programme is reaching the target audience and whether it is cost–effective in relation to the other programmes operated by the organization.

Programme coordinators use information to monitor the progress of the programme in relation to its objectives; to allocate resources; to determine when programme strategies should be modified; and to decide when additional staff training is needed.

Supervisory level staff

Supervisors use information provided by the distributors, or by the administration in the form of feedback, to monitor the performance of the distributors; to perform personal planning conferences; to identify distributors in need of refresher training; and to streamline their supervisory visits.

Community-level staff

Distributors use their own data on users, and feedback from supervisors to monitor their performance in relation to their personal objectives and in comparison with other distributors. Feedback is essential to ensure that distributors understand the importance of data collection.

Distributors also use information gained from observation of and conversations with users to find ways to improve the performance of the programme.

Table 6. Examples of information use at various management levels

Level	Management questions	Suggested indicators	Source of data
Distributor	Has the distributor achieved his or her personal service goal?	Number of users registered; number of contraceptive methods distributed.	Service record forms.
Supervisor	How well are the distributors performing?	Number of users registered; number of contraceptive methods distributed; number of IEC talks given.	Service record forms; receipts from contraceptive sales; observation of distributors during supervisory visits.
Coordinator	What is the most effective use of supervisors' time?	CYP achieved per supervisor; number and duration of supervisory visits.	Supervisors' reports; supervisors' time sheets.
Programme director	Which service-delivery approach works best?	CYP achieved by service modality; level of satisfaction among users.	Programme coordinators' reports; results of user surveys.
Executive committee	Is the CBD programme more cost-effective this year than last, and are the results worth the expense?	Recurrent costs divided by CYP attained, for each year; programme coverage compared with the results of other service-delivery strategies.	Annual budgets; CYP statistics by year; cost per CYP for other service-delivery strategies; survey data on sources of family planning services.
Ministry of Finance or funding agency	Are the funds being spent as planned?	Money spent, by budget category.	Quarterly financial reports.

Estimating the couple–years of protection

Programme managers have often encountered problems in measuring the success of family planning programmes in terms of the numbers of users served because of the difficulty in determining how long and how frequently each registered user has been receiving services.

While no method of measuring service-delivery output is perfect, a practical and useful concept is that of "couple–years of protection". This approach allows the programme manager to measure the impact of the programme in terms of the estimated amount of potential contraceptive protection provided to users. CYP is particularly useful as a standard measure of output for comparing the cost–effectiveness of two or more family planning programmes, even programmes from different countries.

As stated in the *Logistics guidelines for family planning programmes* (United States: Department of Health and Human Services, 1987):

"The CYP index provides a way to determine the total contraceptive protection offered by different methods issued by a programme during a certain time period. One CYP is equal to 12 couple–months of protection, which could be attributed to any person–time combination, from one couple practicing birth control for one year, to 12 couples practicing birth control for one month each. Thus, CYP indicates how much contraceptive protection time could result from the quantity of contraceptives dispensed."

Note, however, that to measure the impact of the programme in terms of the prevalence of contraceptive use in the programme area, a small-scale survey would be required. (For further information about using small-scale surveys, see Nosseir et al., 1984.)

If CYP is used to measure the performance of a programme, the programme manager must ensure that the necessary data are recorded as part of the ongoing monitoring and reporting system. In particular, the number and type of contraceptives given to each acceptor for personal use (i.e. not for redistribution) must be recorded on each occasion. This is relatively simple if begun at the start of the programme. However, reliable data cannot be generated retrospectively.

79

Table 7. Estimating the couple–years of protection

Contraceptive method	Amount distributed (A)	Estimated annual requirements per couple (B)	CYP (A ÷ B)
Oral contraceptives	290 416	13 cycles	22 340
Condoms	193 596	144 pieces	1 344
Foaming tablets	87 221	144 tablets	606
Spermicidal foam or cream	1 116	6 tubes	186

Total CYP = 24 476

To calculate the CYP for each method dispensed through a CBD programme, the quantity of each contraceptive method dispensed to users for personal use should simply be divided by the average quantity of each method used by a couple in one year (see Table 7). The total CYP can then be calculated, as shown in the table.

Evaluating the programme

The purpose of evaluation is to improve the programme. Evaluation is carried out by reviewing and analysing the hypothesis upon which the programme is built and drawing up a set of recommendations for strengthening the design of the programme. Periodic evaluation of the programme will help ensure that it is moving towards its goals in a timely fashion and in as efficient a manner as possible.

This section describes the general concept of evaluation, and then discusses some of the factors that should be considered when evaluating a CBD programme.

How is evaluation different from monitoring and supervision?

Evaluation differs from monitoring and supervision in several ways. First, monitoring and supervision are continuous, ongoing activities, whereas evaluation takes place periodically (e.g. annually or every few years). However, there is some overlap between these activities, since some of the data collected as part of the monitoring and supervision system will be required for evaluating the programme.

Secondly, although evaluators look at many of the same data that programme managers and supervisors collect and use for programme management purposes, the evaluation team will also ask questions whose answers are not normally found in the data generated by the programme's ongoing activities.

For example, the evaluators may wish to measure the relationship between the programme and factors that are external to the programme, such as the impact of the provision of family planning services on infant mortality. Such data are not normally collected by family planning service providers, and therefore will not be included in the programme's management information system. The evaluators would instead rely on data such as demographic or census data recorded by the government department of statistics.

Evaluations may also take place as a result of a special event, such as the completion of a census or a demographic survey that may contain data that can be very useful to the programme.

To ensure that the evaluation focuses on issues useful to the programme, a list of questions should be prepared in advance in collaboration with those who will be responsible for implementing the recommendations that result from the evaluation. Such participation is essential if the evaluation is to result in a strengthened programme.

Since evaluations are not part of a programme's normal activities, and since they are often undertaken by people who are not full-time programme staff, evaluation activities are often viewed with misgivings by programme management. This results from a misconception of the nature and purpose of evaluation. Evaluation should be a collaborative effort between programme management and the evaluation team.

Programme management should also schedule periodic evaluations as part of the programme. Simple techniques, such as sending out one-page questionnaires to distributors, can be used to identify potential problems before they become serious. For example, the distributor can indicate if supply is a problem, if assistance is needed to generate community support, or if there are any unforeseen obstacles to the programme.

When should evaluations be scheduled, and by whom?

Evaluations should be scheduled when sufficient data regarding the impact and performance of the programme have accumulated, or can be generated, upon which meaningful and useful conclusions can be drawn.

As discussed above, programme evaluations are often scheduled by others, in response to needs that are external to the programme. Examples include evaluations that are undertaken at the request of government departments or international donor organizations. Indeed, the scheduling of such evaluations may interfere or conflict with the programme's own schedule.

Programme management should work closely with external evaluation teams to ensure that the evaluation does not inter-

Fig. 21. A checklist for evaluating a CBD programme

1. State clearly the objectives that the programme was supposed to achieve, and how the design was to have increased the likelihood of achieving those objectives. Include assumptions upon which the design was based.

2. Prepare a list of questions to ask in determining the programme's success in meeting its objectives.

3. Identify the kinds and sources of information you need to answer the questions.

4. Compile the information and analyse it in relation to progress made in meeting measurable objectives.

5. Document the factors, negative and positive, that affected the performance of the programme.

6. Prepare an evaluation report that:

   — states the goals and objectives of the programme;
   — describes the findings of the evaluation in terms of measurable achievements and the factors that influenced the achievements;
   — contains a list of recommendations, based on the findings, for improving the programme.

7. Disseminate the findings and recommendations of the report to appropriate staff members and other individuals involved in planning and supervising the programme.

8. Use the report to prepare the next annual (or other periodic) plan for programme activities. On the basis of the findings and recommendations, you may decide to modify the programme, the kinds of data collected, etc.

fere with the programme and that the findings are made available to the programme in the form of feedback.

Evaluation teams should include people who are experts in family planning service delivery, statisticians, and people who can communicate effectively in non-technical language with decision-makers who may not be familiar with evaluation methodology. A checklist for undertaking a programme evaluation is presented in Fig. 21. While the checklist is illustrative, it may be used as a general guide to programme evaluation.

6. Special issues

This chapter addresses six issues of particular relevance to CBD: gaining support from health professionals; legal issues; integrating other health services with family planning; quality assurance; AIDS; and breast-feeding.

This chapter discusses six of the most important CBD-related issues raised by managers, service providers, policy-makers, and researchers. There are many strategies for dealing with these issues, and the questions they raise have no simple answers.

"The doctors in my country are resistant to the idea of community personnel distributing the pill. How can I convince them that the distributors can do a good job?"

"How can I operate a CBD programme when the laws in my country state that only medical personnel can distribute contraceptives?"

"Should we have our mobile immunization team distribute contraceptives, or will we need additional staff devoted just to family planning?"

"How can I ensure the quality of the family planning services we provide?"

"AIDS is a major health problem in my country. How can the CBD programme help?"

"How can a CBD programme help promote breast-feeding as a means of birth spacing?"

Clearly, the answers to these questions are as diverse as the countries and communities which CBD programmes serve. The purpose here is to discuss the issues so that programme managers can make decisions based on their own experience and the specific situation.

84

Gaining support from health professionals

In many countries, community-based programmes that rely on paramedical or community personnel to provide family planning education and distribute contraceptives reflect a significant departure from standard health care delivery.

Many CBD programmes report that they have had to overcome opposition from health professionals who were either concerned about the quality of care that could be provided by non-professionals, or fearful that the CBD programme would intrude in an area which they believed belonged in the hands of doctors and nurses.

Gaining support from health professionals is essential if CBD programmes are to succeed. This may be achieved in several ways. In Kenya, a rural CBD programme has overcome opposition from physicians by employing nursing staff to train its distributors, and requiring that clients receive their initial supplies of contraceptives in a clinic, and have periodic medical check-ups.

In other countries, similar problems have been solved by appointing respected physicians to the medical committee of the CBD programme, where they help set standards for community worker training and ensure appropriate referral of clients to clinics.

In countries or regions where maternal morbidity and mortality are particularly high, it may be useful to inform health professionals of the health benefits of birth spacing to demonstrate that the risks associated with using the family planning methods provided by the CBD programme are insignificant in comparison with the risks women face during pregnancy and childbirth. This fact, along with high-quality training and supervision for distributors, can help win the support of the medical community.

A survey was conducted in Mexico in 1982 to determine whether morbidity and mortality were any higher among users of oral contraceptives in a CBD programme than among women who obtained the pill from other sources (Serrano et al., 1987). The study found that CBD acceptors were as healthy as acceptors from other sources. The increased prevalence of contraceptive use resulting from the introduction of the CBD programme also benefited the women by reducing the incidence of unwanted pregnancy with its associated dangers. Although this study deals with only one locality, it seems likely that the general findings would apply to most CBD programmes.

85

Keys to gaining support from the medical community

- Develop and adhere to medically accepted standards of service delivery to ensure high technical quality.

- Include health professionals in programme decision-making, the training of distributors, and supervision.

- Ask a well respected physician to participate in drawing up a checklist of contraindications to oral contraception for use by distributors.

- Maintain a referral system that will help health personnel understand the benefits of maintaining links between the programme and clinical services.

Addressing legal issues

In some countries, the distribution of contraceptives may be affected by laws and regulations. These laws and regulations usually pertain to three areas (for additional information, see Nkubu, 1987):

1. Public information and advertising of contraceptive products.

2. The importation, manufacture, distribution, sale and use of contraceptives.

3. Categories of agents allowed to distribute contraceptives.

For most CBD programmes, the most common legal or regulatory problem concerns the last area. Oral contraceptives are frequently available only on prescription, which effectively limits their distribution to physicians.

If the distribution of oral contraceptives by trained community workers is a problem, the easiest solution is to arrange for new users to receive their initial prescription from a clinician, with subsequent resupply from the nearest distributor.

Table 8 provides a checklist for analysing the laws and regulations that may affect the distribution of contraceptives.

Where potential barriers exist, their impact on a CBD programme may be reduced by directing the information towards individuals and small groups and by focusing on the importance of family planning and the location of services, rather than on contraceptives *per se*.

86

Table 8. Checklist for analysing laws and regulations that may affect the distribution of contraceptives

Subject	Sources of information
Health policy	
Does the government have a specific policy to reduce infant and maternal deaths?	National health plans. Ratification of international treaties and declarations concerning "Health for All" and other health matters. Statements of high-ranking government officials, such as the Minister of Health.
Human rights	
Has the government signed or issued any documents that:	World Population Plan of Action (1974, amended 1984).
–guarantee individuals the right to choose the number and spacing of their children?	
–guarantee improved rights for women?	Convention on the Elimination of All Forms of Discrimination Against Women (1984).
Information, education and communication	
Is public information about family planning permitted? If so, what media may be used?	Criminal law.
What, if any, restrictions on messages exist?	Obscenity laws.
What restrictions are there on advertising approved prescription contraceptives?	Communications law.
May non-prescription contraceptives be advertised?	Health regulations and codes of ethics.
Distribution of contraceptives	
Is the distribution of contraceptives permitted?	National laws.
Must oral contraceptives be prescribed by a physician? Are physical examinations required?	Guidelines for medical practice.
May oral contraceptives only be dispensed by a pharmacist?	Ministry of Health and pharmaceutical regulations.
What categories of personnel are authorized to distribute oral contraceptives?	Health code.
Are there age requirements for receiving contraceptive services and information?	Family code or minors' code; health code and regulations.
Must the user be married? If so, is spousal consent required?	Often a matter of custom, but sometimes found in regulations of the service provider.

87

Table 8 (continued)

Subject	Sources of information
Are there mechanisms to assure that contraceptives are of satisfactory quality?	Ministry of Health regulations.
Is the price of contraceptives controlled?	Ministry of Health or Finance regulations.
Importation	
Is the importation of contraceptives permitted? Are there taxes or duties on imported contraceptives?	Import and export laws and regulations.
Are there regulations concerning donated products? May they be sold? If so, by whom?	Ministry of Finance (Commerce or Justice); by-laws governing not-for-profit organizations.

Source: Isaacs S. *A checklist for examining laws and regulations affecting family planning.* New York, Columbia University, Center for Population and Family Health, 1988 (unpublished document; available on request from the Center for Population and Family Health, Columbia University, New York, NY 10032, USA).

In some communities, it may be necessary to define intended clients as "married couples" or "women in union", to overcome opposition.

Authorizing community workers to distribute contraceptives may require the following:

—initial prescription by a physician with subsequent distribution at the community level;

—periodic review of distributors' records by an authorizing physician;

—referral of new clients to a clinic for a medical consultation within a specified period after receiving their initial supply of contraceptives;

—referral of clients to clinical sites for oral contraception, as well as IUD insertion and voluntary sterilization.

CBD programmes in many countries have dealt successfully with a variety of legal issues. In Oyo State, Nigeria, CBD programme managers have avoided legal conflicts by involving Ministry of Health officials in planning the programme, issuing certificates of competence to their community workers, and documenting their supervision system.

It is essential that CBD programmes sensitize legislators to the important role of CBD in improving health and contributing to development efforts. In addition, programme managers should consider community sensitivities in designing public information strategies and selecting target groups and should ensure that close links are maintained with clinical health services.

Integrating other health services

There are many reasons why a programme manager may decide that family planning services should be provided by people who are responsible for delivering other community-based health services. These people may already be working in the community, have the confidence of the local population, and require relatively little training (compared with that required by a new community worker) to assume additional tasks.

Supervision and other support systems for the community-based services may already be in place. Furthermore, offering family planning services in conjunction with other health services may increase acceptance of family planning in the community.

On the other hand, there are many reasons why a manager may decide not to combine family planning services with other health services. The requirements for CBD workers to provide information about family planning methods, assess clients for possible contraindications, and identify clients who need to be referred for clinical services may be difficult to meet for health workers who are already responsible for many community health needs.

Other health interventions may involve very different timing and frequency of contact between the community workers and the clients than those involved in CBD. They may also have different target groups from those of the CBD programme, or they may not be well accepted by the CBD target groups.

However, given political and financial constraints, as well as the need for many basic health services in most countries and communities, programme managers may decide to integrate family planning with other community health services. The primary health services with which family planning has most frequently been integrated are those providing oral rehydration therapy, treatment for intestinal parasitic infections or malaria, and immunizations. There are positive and negative aspects of providing CBD with each of these services, as discussed below.

Oral rehydration therapy

The target group of oral rehydration therapy (ORT) programmes – mothers of infants and young children – is the same as that of many CBD programmes. The interventions are relatively simple, and the supplies needed can easily be carried by a community worker. Both CBD and ORT involve educating people to use something that they will continue to use following contact with the health worker, and they both require referral and medical back-up services.

On the other hand, even with adequate training and supervision, errors in the administration of ORT may have serious consequences, which could discredit the CBD programme. Since both ORT and contraceptive use require education of clients, it is also unlikely that appropriate instruction in both could be provided in the same visit.

The client follow-up requirements of CBD programmes are different from those of ORT programmes. Other factors to be considered are the frequency of diarrhoeal disease in the target community, the seasonal variation in the need for ORT, the community's perception of the ORT programme, and the interest of the ORT staff in adding family planning services to their list of responsibilities.

Treatment of parasitic infections

Programme managers who are interested in providing community-based family planning services may decide to combine these services with services providing treatment for parasitic infections. They should recognize, however, that parasite treatment services are usually provided seasonally, rather than regularly throughout the year. Parasite treatment services also tend to focus on screening the entire population, rather than target groups who may be potential users of family planning services. The requirements for follow-up are also different. However, if a successful, well accepted parasite treatment programme exists in communities which are also targets for CBD services, programme managers may consider this option.

Treatment of malaria

Malaria treatment programmes, particularly those that use standard treatment regimens, may also be a possible health service into which CBD can be integrated.

Malaria treatment usually involves providing clients with doses of chloroquine or other antimalarials. Clearly, if the target groups of the malaria treatment and CBD programmes are the same, health workers could deliver both services simultaneously. Treatment programmes that target women and children may at least provide an opportunity for initial contact with women who are potential users of family planning services.

However, as with parasite treatment programmes, malaria treatment services may be provided seasonally according to need rather than continuously, and the main target groups for the CBD programme may form only a small part of the target population for malaria treatment.

Nevertheless, if the malaria treatment programme is well accepted by the community, provides regular services throughout the year, and includes women of reproductive age or their children in its target population, programme managers may consider incorporating family planning services into such programmes.

Immunizations

Of all the community-based health services, immunization programmes probably offer the least opportunity for incorporating family planning. Immunizations must be given on a very strict time schedule, which is unlikely to meet the needs of family planning clients.

None the less, in some circumstances, immunization programmes may provide an opportunity to deliver family planning services. Immunization programmes may be very active, with their staff fully occupied, during the initial immunization campaign, but as their services become necessary only for immigrants and young children, they become much less active. At this stage, the staff could be re-trained as CBD workers. They could combine their family planning activities with identifying people in need of immunization, maintaining vaccination cards, and informing the community of additional immunizations available.

Other health services

Many CBD programmes have found that other basic health services can also be incorporated into their activities. For example, the distributors in a CBD programme in the Dominican Republic provide basic information related to clean water and hygiene, give vaccinations, and treat minor injuries and illnesses.

This strategy is successful because of the close links between the CBD programme and the clinical health services, and because the CBD workers receive continuous training and supervision to develop and maintain their skills in a variety of areas.

Before deciding to integrate family planning with other community-based health services, programme managers should assess the following:

—the similarity of the target groups;

—the compatibility of the provider–client contact schedules;

—the community's acceptance of the health service;

—the willingness and ability of programme staff to take on additional responsibilities;

—the adaptability of the existing management, supervisory, logistics and training systems to the needs of the CBD programme;

—the availability of alternative personnel and support.

Quality assurance

While it is widely recognized that CBD programmes can substantially increase the quantity of family planning services, many health professionals, policy-makers and other influential people (including community leaders) have expressed concern about maintaining the quality of services in the context of CBD.

Service providers in CBD programmes lack the professional training of most clinical staff and have much less supervision. Thus, it is important to monitor several elements of quality that require particular attention in CBD programmes.

In 1989, a working group was set up to consider the issue of measuring quality in family planning programmes. The group, composed of representatives of fifteen international organizations involved in family planning, concluded that there are six broad elements that contribute to service quality (Subcommittee on Quality Indicators in Family Planning Service Delivery, 1989). Each of these elements is relevant to CBD programmes.

Choice of family planning methods

Programmes should offer clients a variety of family planning methods, and ensure that those methods are always available. CBD programmes may provide barrier methods and oral contraceptives, methods which may be appropriate for users with very different needs. In addition, they may refer clients for other methods that are not available directly from the programme, such as voluntary sterilization, injectables, IUDs and natural methods of family planning.

Information and counselling

CBD programmes should be particularly careful about the information given to clients. Several studies of CBD programmes have noted that some distributors often omit important information during their contacts with clients, while others give inaccurate or confusing information. Programme managers should ensure that all clients are given information about:

- The range of family planning methods available, both directly from the CBD programme and by referral, together with their contraindications, advantages and disadvantages.

- The proper use of the method selected, including its potential side-effects and the possible impact on the client's fertility or sex life.

- The procedures for and frequency of resupply of contraceptives, the availability of counselling, referral services, etc. (Bruce, 1989).

The information given to clients should be complete, without being too detailed, to ensure that clients fully understand the methods that are available. It should be presented in an unbiased manner to ensure that the decision to use a particular method of family planning is made voluntarily, without undue influence from the distributor.

While it is essential that clients receive this information, it is equally important that they are encouraged to ask questions and to discuss their concerns, fears, reproductive intentions (desire for more children), and other matters that affect use of family planning. Training of CBD workers should include skills in counselling, which will enable them to meet their clients' personal needs and circumstances.

Technical competence

While most family planning programmes acknowledge the importance of technical competence of clinical personnel, it is equally important to ensure the competence of CBD workers. The programme should determine exactly what tasks the CBD worker is expected to do (e.g. provide information, assist clients with making decisions regarding contraception, distribute contraceptives, and make referrals) and then provide training, specific protocols, and supervision to ensure that each worker is capable of performing these tasks.

Interpersonal relations

How clients feel about the services they receive can determine whether or not they continue to use the programme's services and even whether or not they continue to use a particular method of family planning.

It is often difficult to assess relationships between service providers working in community settings and their clients because staff usually work alone. Nevertheless, CBD programmes should encourage their workers to establish and maintain a relationship with their clients based on respect, understanding and honesty. Perhaps the most important element in good communications skills is the ability to listen carefully.

The distributor's tasks should be structured to permit sufficient time to be spent with individual clients. Supervisory visits should be scheduled to allow supervisors to observe distributors communicating with users and to assist the distributor in developing additional communications skills, particularly listening skills.

Mechanisms to encourage continuity

CBD programmes should promote continuity of contraceptive use in the community. This may be done in several ways:

- Clients who have chosen a particular contraceptive method should be able to continue using that method, through easy access to resupply, information about side-effects, etc., as long as that method is appropriate to their personal needs and reproductive intentions.

- Clients whose needs or reproductive intentions have changed should be offered other methods (e.g. clients using oral contraceptives who decide they do not want another child should be advised about the option of voluntary surgical contraception).

- In communities with other family planning services, clients should be supported in their decision to acquire a contraceptive method from another source (e.g. a retail outlet or the private sector). Ideally, the CBD programme should also maintain contact with these clients to assist them with additional information about family planning.

Organization of services

How the programme organizes its services is an important determinant of quality. The quality of the programme will depend on numerous variables that must be monitored to detect whether they have a positive or a negative impact on client satisfaction. These variables include:

The number and variety of services offered:

- Does the distributor offer a variety of methods and brands, and are they locally known and popular?

- Are other family planning services offered through referral?

- Are services other than family planning offered?

- How reliable is the supply of contraceptives?

Accessibility of services:

- Is the distribution site conveniently located and close to other services, such as markets and banks?

- Is the location considered safe by the distributor and the clients?

- What do clients think of the travel time and distance to reach the services?

- Do distributors make house calls?

- Are the opening-times convenient for clients?

- Is there a long wait for service?
- Are fees for service reasonable considering the economic status of the clients?

Appearance of site:

- Is the distribution point relatively attractive, well organized, and comfortable for clients?

Confidentiality:

- Are services provided with respect for client confidentiality?

HIV/AIDS

By 1994, more than 980 000 cases of AIDS had been reported to WHO from over 180 countries and territories (WHO, 1994c). In the face of this growing problem, health professionals and government leaders throughout the world have been looking for ways to prevent the spread of HIV/AIDS. Several strategies have been employed, including the provision of educational and counselling services and the promotion of condom use during sexual intercourse.

As the number of cases of AIDS increases and as public awareness grows, programmes must prepare for a surge in clients seeking information about HIV/AIDS and condoms. Of all family planning service-delivery strategies, CBD promises to have the most to contribute to the prevention of AIDS, since in order to reduce the spread of the disease, information and condoms will have to be distributed far beyond the reach of clinic-based services.

In addition, CBD distributors have access to the community, are aware of local values and cultural mores, and are accepted by the public. This is vitally important for disseminating the AIDS prevention message. In particular, distributors can provide valuable assistance in designing acceptable messages and effective outreach strategies. Since distributors communicate directly with clients about sexual matters, they may also be able to influence their clients' sexual behaviour.

However, managers must consider the potential risks of involving their CBD programmes in AIDS issues. It is particularly important to avoid conveying the impression that AIDS and family planning are somehow linked. Similarly, users must

Table 9. Guidelines for preventing AIDS through CBD programmes

Activity

1. Educate supervisors and distributors about HIV/AIDS, stressing how it is, and how it is not, acquired. Reassure distributors about the negligible risk of acquiring the infection from their clients.

2. Train distributors and supervisors in AIDS education and "safe sex" counselling techniques.

3. Ensure that sufficient condoms are on hand for the additional demand that may be anticipated.

4. Develop referral procedures for clients seeking AIDS-related medical attention, and inform supervisors and distributors about the procedures and confidentiality.

5. Explore the possibility of providing CBD services in the workplace, in order to reach sexually active men more effectively.

6. Recruit supervisors and community volunteers to assist in designing educational materials for clients.

7. Limit AIDS-related activities to education, prevention and referral.

CBD programmes should not:
1. Involve distributors in attempting to diagnose or treat AIDS.
2. Force distributors to participate in AIDS prevention services.

not feel that by visiting the distributor, they are perceived by the public as possibly having AIDS.

It is also important not to overburden CBD workers by giving them other tasks, particularly when there is a possibility that these tasks could become more visible and time-consuming than their family planning work (see Table 9).

If AIDS is a major problem in the area and no prevention campaign exists, however, programme managers should consider postponing family planning activities and allocating the resources to the prevention of AIDS.

Breast-feeding

Breast-feeding is vital for both child survival and family planning. Besides providing nutritional and immunological benefits, breast-feeding makes an important contribution to child spacing in many countries around the world.

Several breast-feeding practices have been found to have a positive impact on child survival and child spacing. To support

97

these practices, CBD programmes should encourage mothers:

- To begin breast-feeding as soon as possible after the child is born.
- To breast-feed exclusively until the baby is 4–6 months old.
- To breast-feed whenever the infant is hungry, day and night.
- To continue to breast-feed when the baby is ill.
- To avoid using feeding-bottles or dummies.
- To continue to breast-feed when other fluids or semi-solid foods are first introduced.

In addition, CBD programmes should ensure that women who are breast-feeding have access to appropriate complementary family planning methods when they are no longer protected against pregnancy.

Fig. 22 provides a decision tree which can be used by CBD programmes to determine whether a breast-feeding woman is protected from pregnancy.

Women who breast-feed experience a natural period of infertility during the early postpartum months. A breast-feeding woman who does not feed her baby foods other than breast milk, is not yet menstruating, and is less than 6 months postpartum has a less than 2% probability of becoming pregnant. The risk of pregnancy increases over time, however, and with decreased frequency of breast-feeding and supplementation with foods other than breast milk (Fig. 22). Breast-feeding does not delay the return to ovulation indefinitely, and most women who breast-feed for longer than 12 months will experience a return to menses before they stop breast-feeding. Breast-feeding women who desire continued protection from pregnancy should begin using an appropriate complementary contraceptive (WHO, 1994d).

If, through the use of this decision tree, it is determined that the woman needs complementary family planning to avoid pregnancy, she should be encouraged to use a method that will not interfere with breast-feeding.

Non-hormonal methods are most appropriate for these women. However, progestogen-only methods may be given to women who prefer oral contraceptives, injectables or implants. Pills containing estrogen (combined oral contraceptives) should be avoided until the child is at least 6 months of age and beginning to take other fluids or semi-solid food (Labbok et al., 1992).

98

Fig. 22. Decision tree for determining whether a breast-feeding woman is protected from pregnancy

Is the client breast-feeding?

YES → Is the client menstruating?
Is the client giving food supplements in addition to breast-feeding?
Has the client been breast-feeding for more than six months?

ALL "NO" → The client is adequately protected from pregnancy

Does the client wish to adopt a contraceptive method to complement breast-feeding, or is she unlikely to return for services?

NO → Advise the client that she may be adequately protected from pregnancy but should return for contraception as soon as one of the three criteria above is not met

YES → Is the client more than six weeks postpartum?

NO → Discuss the suitability of:
– barrier methods

YES → Discuss the suitability of:
– barrier methods
– progestogen-only methods
– IUDs
– injectables

ONE OR MORE "YES" → The client is not adequately protected from pregnancy and requires a complementary method

NO → Does the client desire a method that does not require frequent use or resupply?

YES → Discuss the suitability of:
– IUDs
– injectables

NO → Is the client at risk of circulatory disease?

YES → Discuss the suitability of:
– barrier methods
– progestogen-only methods
– natural family planning

NO → Discuss the suitability of:
– barrier methods
– combined oral contraceptives
– natural family planning
– injectables

WHO 93255

99

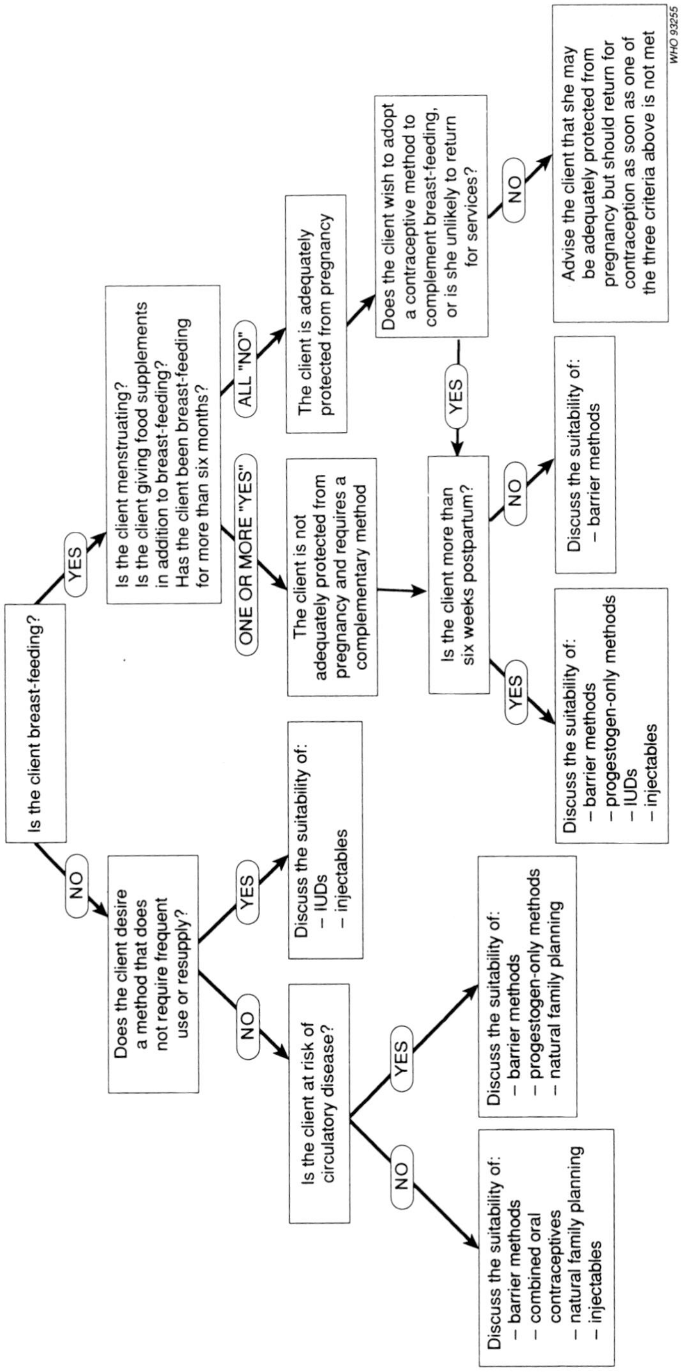

There is evidence that HIV infection can be transmitted to infants through breast-feeding. However, in settings where the primary causes of infant deaths are infectious disease and malnutrition, WHO recommends that breast-feeding should remain the standard advice to pregnant women, including those who are known to be HIV-infected, since in these settings, the advantages of breast-feeding, even for a baby whose mother is HIV-infected, outweigh the risks associated with bottle-feeding. On the other hand, in settings where infectious diseases are not the primary causes of death during infancy, WHO recommends that pregnant women known to be infected with HIV should be advised not to breast-feed but to use a safe feeding alternative for their babies. Women whose infection status is unknown should be advised to breast-feed (Piot et al., 1992).

Clearly, the CBD programme should maintain close links with maternal and child health programmes in the community. Recommendations regarding breast-feeding practices, the introduction of family planning methods after childbirth, and breast-feeding by HIV-positive mothers should not be contradictory and should be reinforced by the various programmes.

This may also be an opportunity for referral to other services: the CBD programme may refer women who are breast-feeding to a breast-feeding support group, which in turn, may refer women to the CBD programme to receive appropriate advice on family planning.

References

BRUCE J (1989) *Fundamental elements of the quality of care: a simple framework.* New York, The Population Council (unpublished document; available on request from The Population Council, 1 Dag Hammarskjold Plaza, New York, NY 10017, USA).

FINCANCIOGLY N (1984) Taking family planning to the people. *Draper Fund report,* 13: 6–8.

LABBOK M ET AL. (1992) *Guidelines for breast-feeding in family planning and child survival programs.* Georgetown, DE, Georgetown University, Institute for Reproductive Health.

NKUBA H (1987) Overview of the legal obstacles to CBD of contraceptives in sub-Saharan Africa. In: *Proceedings of a conference on community-based distribution and alternative delivery systems in Africa, Harare, Zimbawe, November 3–7 1986.* Washington, DC, Public Health Association: 38–42.

NOSSEIR N ET AL. (1984) *The use of mini-surveys for evaluating community-based health interventions.* Paper presented at the Annual Conference of the National Council for International Health, Washington, DC, 11–13 June 1984. Cairo, Social Research Center, The American University; Baltimore, Johns Hopkins Population Center, The Johns Hopkins University.

OAKLEY P (1989) *Community involvement in health development. An examination of the critical issues.* Geneva, World Health Organization.

PACT (1986) *The cost–effectiveness analysis field manual.* New York, NY, Robert Nathan Associates (unpublished document; available on request from PACT, 777 United Nations Plaza, New York, NY 10017, USA).

PIOT P ET AL. (1992) *AIDS in Africa: a manual for physicians.* Geneva, World Health Organization.

REYNOLDS J, GASPARI KC (1986) *Operations research methodologies: cost–effectiveness analysis.* Bethesda, MD, Center for Human Services (PRICOR Monograph Series, Methods Paper 2).

ROSENFIELD A (1986) The medical rationale for CBD strategies. In: *Proceedings of a conference on community-based distribution and alternative delivery systems in Africa, Harare, Zimbabwe, November 3–7 1986.* Washington, DC, Public Health Association.

SAI F (1986) Family planning and maternal health care: a common goal. *World health forum,* 7: 315–324.

SATHAR ZA, CHIDAMBARAM VC (1984) *Differentials in contraceptive use.* Voorburg, International Statistical Institute (WFS Comparative Studies No. 36).

SERRANO A ET AL. (1987) Reproductive risks in a community-based distribution programme of oral contraceptives, Matamoros, Mexico. *Studies in family planning,* 18: 284–290.

SUBCOMMITTEE on QUALITY INDICATORS IN FAMILY PLANNING SERVICE DELIVERY (1989) *Draft report submitted to the USAID Task Force on Standardization of Family Planning Performance Indicators.* New York, The Population Council (unpublished document; available on request from The Population Council, 1 Dag Hammarskjold Plaza, New York, NY 10017, USA).

TERBORGH A ET AL. (1990) *A model of training and quality control in community-based family planning programs.* Arlington, VA, Development Associates Inc.

UNFPA (1991) *Contraceptive requirements and demand for contraceptive commodities in developing countries in the 1990s.* New York, United Nations Population Fund.

UNITED STATES: DEPARTMENT OF HEALTH AND HUMAN SERVICES (1987) *Logistics guidelines for family planning programs.* Atlanta, GA, Centers for Disease Control, National Institutes of Health (available on request from Centers for Disease Control and Prevention, Division of Reproductive Health, Program Services and Development Branch, 1600 Clifton Road NE, Atlanta, GA 30333, USA).

UNITED STATES: DEPARTMENT OF HEALTH AND HUMAN SERVICES (1993) *Logistics guidelines for family planning programs.* Atlanta, GA, Centers for Disease Control and Prevention, National Institutes of Health (available on request from Centers for Disease Control and Prevention, Division of Reproductive Health, Program Services and Development Branch, 1600 Clifton Road NE, Atlanta, GA 30333, USA).

WHO (1994a) *Specification and guidelines for condom procurement by WHO Global Programme on AIDS.* Geneva, World Health Organization (unpublished document; available on request from the Global Programme on AIDS, World Health Organization, 1211 Geneva 27, Switzerland).

WHO (1994b) *Managing condom supply manual.* Geneva, World Health Organization (unpublished draft document; available on request from the Global Programme on AIDS, World Health Organization, 1211 Geneva 27, Switzerland).

WHO (1994c) *Weekly epidemiological record,* **69** (26): 189.

WHO (1994d) *Contraceptive method mix. Guidelines for policy and service delivery.* Geneva, World Health Organization.

Selected further reading

ALTMAN DL, PIOTROW PT (1980) Social marketing: does it work? *Population reports*, Series J, No. 21.

BERTRAND JT ET AL. (1980) Characteristics of successful distributors in the community-based distribution of contraceptives in Guatemala. *Studies in family planning*, 11: 274–285.

BERTRAND JT, MANGANI N, MANSILU M (1984) The acceptability of household distribution of contraceptives in Zaire. *International family planning perspectives*, 10: 21–26.

BHATIA S ET AL. (1980) The Matlab Family Planning–Health Services Project. *Studies in family planning*, 11: 202–212.

BLACKBURN R, KAK N (1987) *Preventing the spread of AIDS in less developed countries: lessons learned from family planning outreach programs*. Paper presented at the 115th meeting of the American Public Health Association, New Orleans, LA, 12–18 October 1987. (Unpublished document PIP/045016; available on request from the Population Information Program, The Johns Hopkins University School of Hygiene and Public Health, 527 St Paul Place, Baltimore, MD 21202, USA.)

BURKHART MC (1981) Issues in community-based distribution of contraceptives. *Pathpapers*, No. 8: 21–37.

CASH RA (1985) *Oral rehydration for the treatment of diarrhea: its value as a health component in community-based family planning distribution programs*. Paper presented at the Workshop on Family Planning and Health Components in Community-Based Distribution (CBD) Projects, Charlottesville, VA, 12–14 January 1982. In: Wawer MJ et al., eds. *Health and family planning in community-based distribution projects*. Boulder, CO, Westview Press: 121–143.

CERANDA GP, HUANG T (1970) Training field workers for family planning. In: Ceranda GP, ed. *Taiwan family planning reader: how a program works*. Taichung, Chinese Center for International Training in Family Planning: 45–63.

CHEN KHM, WORTH G (1982) *Cost–effectiveness of a community-based family planning program in Cheju, Korea.* Paper presented at the International Health Conference, Washington, DC, 14–16 June 1982. (Unpublished document PIP/008954; available on request from the Population Information Program, The Johns Hopkins University, Baltimore, MD 21202, USA.)

COLUMBIA UNIVERSITY: CENTER FOR POPULATION AND FAMILY HEALTH (1981) *New strategies for the delivery of maternal/ child health and family planning services in rural and semi-urban slum areas of Mexico.* New York.

CUCA R, PIERCE CS (1977) Experimentation in family planning and delivery systems: an overview. *Studies in family planning,* 8: 302–310.

DUHL LJ (1984) Social communication, organization, and community development: family planning in Thailand. (Unpublished document PIP/037629; available on request from the Population Information Program, The Johns Hopkins University, Baltimore, MD 21202, USA.)

ECONOMIC AND SOCIAL COMMISSION FOR ASIA AND THE PACIFIC (ESCAP) (1984) *Inventory of selected local family planning programme experiences in countries of the ESCAP region, Volume IV.* New York, United Nations.

EDMUNDS M, STRACHAN D, VRIESENDORP S (1987) *Client-responsive family planning: a handbook for providers.* Watertown, MA, The Pathfinder Fund.

EL TOM AR (1982) The Sudan community-based health and family planning project: description of a training course. Paper presented at the International Health Conference, Washington, DC, 14–16 June 1982. In: Wawer MJ et al., eds. *Health and family planning in community-based distribution projects.* Boulder, CO, Westview Press: 417–422.

EL TOM AR ET AL. (1984) Developing the skills of illiterate health workers. *World health forum,* 5: 216–220.

EL TOM AR ET AL. (1987) Community and individual acceptance: family planning services in the Sudan. New York, Columbia University, Center for Population and Family Health (CPFH Working Paper No. 14): 12–30.

EL TOM AR, LAURO D (1984) *Phasing the introduction of MCH/FP services: the Sudan community-based family health project.* Paper presented at the International Health Conference, Washington, DC, June 1984. (Unpublished document PNAAY-515; available on request from Development

Information Services Clearinghouse, Suite 1010, 1500 Wilson Boulevard, Arlington, VA 22209-2404, USA.)

FAMILY PLANNING ASSOCIATION OF SRI LANKA: EVALUATION AND RESEARCH DIVISION (1982) *Mithuri user survey.* Colombo.

FAMILY PLANNING PRIVATE SECTOR (FPPS) PROGRAMME: KENYA (1989) *FPPS community-based distribution programme record-keeping procedures.* (Unpublished document; available on request from John Snow Inc., 1616 N. Fort Myer Drive, 11th floor, Arlington, VA 22209, USA.)

FOREIT JR ET AL. (1978) Community-based and commercial contraceptive distribution: an inventory and appraisal. *Population reports*, Series J, No. 19.

FOREIT JR, FOREIT K (1984) Quarterly versus monthly supervision of CBD family planning programs: an experimental study in northeast Brazil. *Studies in family planning*, 15: 112–120.

GADALLA S, NASSER N, GILLESPIE DG (1980) Household distribution of contraceptives in rural Egypt. *Studies in family planning*, 11: 105–113.

GILLESPIE DG (1985) Issues in integrated family planning and health programs. Paper presented at the Workshop on Family Planning and Health Components in Community-Based Distribution (CBD) Projects, Charlottesville, VA, 12–14 January 1982. In: Wawer MJ et al., eds. *Health and family planning in community-based distribution projects.* Boulder, CO, Westview Press: 25–41.

GOLDEN AS, WAWER MJ, MERCER MA (1985) Training CBD workers for family planning and health interventions. Paper presented at the Workshop on Family Planning and Health Components in Community-Based Distribution (CBD) Projects, Charlottesville, VA, 12–14 January 1982. In: Wawer MJ et al., eds. *Health and family planning in community-based distribution projects.* Boulder, CO, Westview Press: 385–406.

GOVERNMENT OF SENEGAL: MINISTRY OF HEALTH & UNITED STATES AGENCY FOR INTERNATIONAL DEVELOPMENT (1982) *Evaluation conjointe final (Gouvernement du Sénégal—Ministère de la Santé publique — Agence pour le Développement International des Etats Unis) du projet de développement de service de santé rural au Sine Saloum. [Joint end of project evaluation of the Rural Health Service Development Project at Sine Saloum.* (Unpublished document PD-ABA-583; available from Development Information Services Clearinghouse, Suite 1010, 1500 Wilson Boulevard, Arlington, VA 22209-2404, USA.)

HOEY JM, ARYAL S, THAPA R (1981) Building the supervision system: experiences from Nepal. In: Campbell JM, ed. *The training and support of primary health care workers. Proceedings of the 1981 International Health Conference, Washington, DC, 15–17 June 1981.* Washington, DC, National Council for International Health: 195–200.

HUBER SC ET AL. (1975) Contraceptive distribution—taking supplies to villages and households. *Population reports,* Series J, No. 5.

KOLS AJ, WAWER MJ (1982) Community-based health and family planning. *Population reports,* Series L-3, 10 (6).

LECOMTE J ET AL. (1982) *An evaluation of the population and family planning support project in Morocco.* (Unpublished document PD-AAL-080; available on request from Development Information Services Clearinghouse, Suite 1010, 1500 Wilson Boulevard, Arlington, VA 22209-2404, USA.)

MCMAHON R ET AL. (1992) *On being in charge: a guide to management in primary health care,* 2nd ed. Geneva, World Health Organization.

ORY HW, FORREST J, LINCOLN R (1983) *Making choices: evaluating the health risks and benefits of birth control methods.* New York, Alan Guttmacher Institute.

OSBORN RW, REINKE WA (1981) *Community-based distribution of contraception: a review of field experience.* Baltimore, MD, Johns Hopkins Population Center, The Johns Hopkins University, School of Hygiene and Public Health.

PARKER RL (1985) Selected health components of community-based distribution programs. Paper presented at the Workshop on Family Planning and Health Components in Community-Based Distribution (CBD) Projects, Charlottesville, VA, 12–14 January 1982. In: Wawer MJ et al., eds. *Health and family planning in community-based distribution projects.* Boulder, CO, Westview Press: 333–363.

PHILLIPS JF ET AL. (1982) The demographic impact of the family planning – health services project in Matlab, Bangladesh. *Studies in family planning,* 13: 131–140.

PYLE DF (1984) *Management in a successful community-based services program in Bangladesh.* (Unpublished document PIP/025292; available on request from the Population Information Program, The Johns Hopkins University, 527 St Paul Place, Baltimore, MD 21202, USA.)

RAMOS M ET AL. (1986) *An experiment to improve an IUD insertion and medical back-up component of a community-based distribution program in Lima, Peru.* Paper presented at the Annual Meeting of the American Public Health Association, Las Vegas, NV, 28 September–3 October 1986. (Unpublished document CPFH/20801cr986; available on request from the Center for Communication Programs, The Johns Hopkins University, 527 St Paul Place, Baltimore, MD 21202, USA.)

ROSENFIELD A (1971) Family planning: an expanded role for paramedical personnel. *American journal of obstetrics and gynecology,* 110: 1030–1039.

ROSENFIELD A (1974) Auxiliaries and family planning. *Lancet,* i: 443–445.

ROSENFIELD AG, MAINE D, GOROSH ME (1980) Nonclinical distribution of the pill in the developing world. *International family planning perspectives,* 6: 130–135.

ROSS JA (1985) *Family planning pilot projects in Africa: review and synthesis.* New York, International Bank for Reconstruction and Development (World Bank PHN Technical Note 85–7).

SIRAGELDIN I, SALKEVER D, OSBORN R, EDS. (1983) *Evaluating family planning programs: international experience with cost–effectiveness analysis and cost–benefit analysis.* Proceedings of the International Workshop on Cost–Effectiveness Analysis and Cost–Benefit Analysis in Family Planning Programs, St Michaels, MD, 17–20 August 1981. New York, NY, St Martins Press.

WAWER MJ ET AL., EDS. (1985) *Health and family planning in community-based distribution programmes.* Boulder, CO, Westview Press.

WAWER MJ, MERCER MA (1982) *The training of workers for community-based family planning and health projects.* Baltimore, MD, The Johns Hopkins University, School of Hygiene and Public Health.

WESTOFF CF, OCHOA LH (1991) *Unmet need and the demand for family planning.* Columbia, MD, Macro International Inc., Institute for Resource Development (Demographic and Health Surveys Comparative Studies No. 5).

WORTMAN J (1975) Training nonphysicians in family planning services. *Population reports,* No. 6: J89.

Annex 1. Projected demand for contraceptives in developing countries, by method, 1990–2000

Year	Estimated no. of cycles of pills (in millions)	Estimated no. of condoms (in millions)	Estimated no. of injectables (in thousands)	Estimated no. of IUDs (in thousands)	Estimated no. of voluntary sterilization procedures (in thousands)		
					Total	Female	Male
1990	685	3 412	49 452	26 442	11 947	9 870	2 077
1991	708	3 604	51 938	27 143	12 497	10 329	2 168
1992	732	3 797	54 425	27 843	13 048	10 788	2 260
1993	755	3 989	56 911	28 544	13 599	11 247	2 352
1994	778	4 181	59 398	29 245	14 150	11 706	2 444
1995	801	4 373	61 884	29 945	14 700	12 165	2 535
1996	866	4 547	66 465	31 101	15 309	12 626	2 683
1997	931	4 721	71 046	32 256	15 917	13 087	2 830
1998	996	4 894	75 626	33 412	16 526	13 549	2 977
1999	1 061	5 068	80 207	34 568	17 134	14 010	3 124
2000	1 126	5 242	84 788	35 723	17 743	14 471	3 272
Total	9 439	47 828	712 140	336 222	162 570	133 848	28 722

Source: *Contraceptive requirements and demand for contraceptive commodities in developing countries in the 1990s.* New York, United Nations Population Fund, 1991.

109

Annex 2. Sources of demographic data for planning CBD programmes

In most countries, the best source of demographic data for programme planning and evaluation purposes is the national office responsible for collecting and analysing census and vital statistical data. Although it varies from country to country, this office is often located within the Ministry of Planning or in an independent institute of statistics.

Alternatively, data may be obtained from the Demographic and Health Surveys (DHS) programme, which was developed with support from the United States Agency for International Development (USAID) to assist developing countries in carrying out population and health surveys. For further information, contact the Institute for Resource Development at the address below.

Demographic and Health Surveys (DHS)
Macro International Inc.
Institute for Resource Development
Suite 4000
8850 Stanford Boulevard
Columbia, MD 21045
USA

Other sources

Centers for Disease Control and Prevention (CDC)
Division of Reproductive Health
Behavioral, Epidemiology, and Demographic
Research Branch
Atlanta, GA 30333
USA

The Population Council
1 Dag Hammarskjold Plaza
New York, NY 10017
USA

Population Reference Bureau
1875 Connecticut Avenue N.W.
Washington, DC 30009
USA

United Nations
Statistical Office
2 United Nations Plaza
New York, NY 10017
USA

United Nations Population Fund (UNFPA)
220 East 42nd Street
New York, NY 10017
USA

Annex 3. A sample community survey of fertility and use of family planning methods among women of reproductive age (15–45 years)

Organization: _____

Interview record form

	Numbers of visits to household				
	1	2	3	4	5
Date of interview					
Name of interviewer					
Duration of interview (minutes)					
Language of interview					
Result[a]					
Date and time of next appointment					

[a] 1: Interview completed. 2: Interview partly completed – appointment made to complete interview. 3: Appointment made for interview later. 4: Refusal: no interview obtained. 5: No one at home. 6: Eligible respondent not at home. 7: No eligible respondent(s). 8: Other (specify).

Identification of respondent

Cluster no. _____   Area no. _____
Household no. _____   Respondent no. _____

Introducing yourself

Introduce yourself in the following manner when you first call at the designated household:

"How do you do? I am (name) _____. The (name of organization) _____ is conducting a survey on the need for family planning services in your community. I have several questions to ask you. I know you are very busy, but it will not take very long, and I would appreciate it very much if you would help us by answering these questions.

I assure you that your answers will be kept confidential and used solely for research purposes.

First, I would like to know how many people are living in this household, then we will move on to several other questions."

_____ (Number) in household

A. Background characteristics of respondent

A.1 In what month and year were you born? _____

A.2 How old were you on your last birthday? _____ Years

A.3 Have you ever attended school? _____ Yes _____ No

If yes, what was the highest level of school you attended?

_____ Primary _____ Middle _____ Secondary

_____ College/University

If no, can you read a letter or newspaper easily, with difficulty, or not at all?

_____ Easily _____ With difficulty _____ Not at all

A.4 What is the average monthly income (in local currency) of your family?

B. Marital status and fertility

B.1   What is your current marital status?

_____ Single _____ Married _____ Divorced

_____ Widowed _____ Separated

B.2   Have you ever been pregnant?

_____ Yes _____ No (go to question C.1)

B.3   How many children have you given birth to, including those who may have survived only briefly? _____

B.4   When was your last child born?

_____ Month _____ Year, or _____ Age

B.5   Did you breast-feed your last child at all?

_____ Yes _____ No (go to question B.7)

B.6   Are you still breast-feeding?

_____ Yes _____ No _____ Child died

If you are not still breast-feeding, for how long did you breast-feed your last child? _____ (months)

B.7   Have your periods returned?

_____ Yes _____ No

B.8   Have you had a period in the last four weeks?

_____ Yes (go to question C.4) _____ No

B.9   Are you pregnant now?

_____ Yes _____ No _____ Not sure

B.10 Judging from your partner's and your physical condition, can you become pregnant whenever you want to?

_____ Yes _____ No _____ Not sure

If no or not sure, why?

_____ Because partner has been sterilized

_____ Because respondent has been sterilized

_____ Other reason (specify)

B.11 Do you want to have (more) children?

_____ Yes _____ No _____ Not sure

If yes, how long do you want to wait before having the (next) child? _____ (months)

C. Knowledge and attitude to contraception, and use of contraceptives

C.1 Do you know about any methods that are used to prevent women from getting pregnant too often or having more children than they want? (*Interviewer: do not suggest any methods.)

_____ Yes _____No (go to question D.8)

C.2 What methods do you know about? (Note down any methods mentioned in column 1 of Table 1.)

C.3 Have you ever used any of the methods we have talked about?

_____ Yes _____ No (go to question C.7)

If yes, which were these? (Tick in column 2 of Table 1.)

C.4 Are you currently using any method?

_____ Yes _____ No

Table 1. Record of knowledge and history of use of contraception

Method	Knowledge of method (see question C.2)	History of use (see question C.3)	Preferred method (see question C.9)
Condom			
Sponge			
Foams, creams, jellies and vaginal suppositories			
Diaphragm			
Oral contraceptive pill			
Injectables			
Intrauterine device (IUD)			
Tubal ligation			
Vasectomy			
Rhythm (safe period)			
Withdrawal			
Induced abortion or menstrual regulation			
Avoidance of sexual intercourse			
Other (specify)			

C.5   If yes, which method?

_____

C.6   If no, what was the main reason you stopped using it?

_____   to become pregnant

_____   method failed

_____   infrequent sex

_____   partner disapproved

_____   health concerns

_____   method not available

_____ cost

_____ inconvenience

_____ other (specify)

_____ don't know

(*Check questions B.10 and C.4: if either partner is steri-lized or currently using any method, go to question D.1.)

C.7 What is the main reason that you are not using a method to avoid pregnancy?

_____ want to become pregnant

_____ infrequent sex

_____ postpartum/breast-feeding

_____ menopause/subfecund

_____ lack of knowledge

_____ difficult access to methods

_____ religious beliefs

_____ opposition of partner

_____ fear of side-effects

_____ opposed to family planning

_____ other (specify)

_____ don't know

C.8 Do you intend to use another method to avoid pregnancy at any time in the future?

_____ Yes _____ No (go to question D.1)

_____ Don't know (go to question D.1)

C.9 Which method would you prefer to use? (Tick in column 3 of Table 1.)

C.10 Do you intend to use that method in the next 12 months?

_____ Yes _____ No _____ Don't know

D. Perceived availability and accessibility of sources of contraceptive supplies

D.1 Do you know where to get contraceptive supplies?

_____ Yes _____ No (go to question F.1)

D.2 Where is that? (Tick all places mentioned.)

_____ Health centre

_____ Pharmacy

_____ Traditional healer

_____ Distribution post

_____ Private physician

_____ Hospital

_____ Other (specify)

D.3 If you wanted to obtain contraceptives, which of these places would you prefer to go to? (Note only the first place mentioned.)

D.4 How long would it take you to get there if you went there directly?

_____ minutes _____ hours

D.5 Is that place convenient or inconvenient?

_____ Convenient _____ Inconvenient

_____ Don't know

D.6 Are the staff there helpful or not?

_____ Helpful _____ Not helpful _____ Don't know

D.7 Are the opening-hours convenient?

_____ Yes _____ No _____ Don't know

D.8 Are the costs reasonable?

_____ Yes _____ No _____ Don't know

D.9 What contraceptive methods are available there? (Note all the methods mentioned.)

_____ Condoms

_____ Sponge

_____ Foams, creams, jellies and vaginal suppositories

_____ Diaphragm

_____ Oral contraceptive pill

_____ Injectables

_____ Intrauterine device (IUD)

_____ Tubal ligation

_____ Vasectomy

_____ Induced abortion or menstrual regulation

_____ Other (specify)

D.10 Do the staff there favour any particular methods?

_____ Yes _____ No _____ Don't know

If yes, which one? _____

E. Concluding the interview

E.1 Conclude the interview by saying: "Thank you very much. You have been very helpful. Is there anything you would like to add?"_____

_____

_____

Annex 4. A sample workplan for a CBD programme

Objective: "To establish a community-based distribution (CBD) programme that will provide contraceptive services and information to an estimated 4000 low-income women over the course of one year (1993)."

Activity or task	1	2	3	4	5	6	7	8	9	10	11	12	Personnel responsible
1. Identify local sources of contraceptives and set up supply contracts.	×												Director, coordinator, medical director
2. Hire and train a second coordinator.	×												Director, coordinator
3. Design and pretest information, education and communication (IEC) materials.	×	×											Outside consultant
4. Inform department heads of the plans for the CBD programme and meet to discuss their suggestions.	×												Director, coordinators
5. Select the communities in which to establish the CBD programme.	×		×	×	×	×	×	×	×	×	×	×	Director, coordinators
6. Contact and consult community leaders.	×		×	×	×	×	×	×	×	×	×	×	Director, coordinators
7. Establish an advisory team.	×												Director
8. Hire and train 10 supervisors.	×												Coordinators

Monthly activity schedule

9. Recruit 200 distributors.	×	×	×	×	×	×	×	×	×	×	×	Supervisors, coordinators
10. Train the distributors in family planning counselling and record-keeping.	×		×		×		×		×		×	Training consultant, supervisors
11. Set up a logistics system; receive, document and store the contraceptives.	×	×	×	×	×	×	×	×	×	×	×	Storeroom manager, administrative assistant
12. Supply the distributors with contraceptives and IEC materials.	×	×	×	×	×	×	×	×	×	×	×	Supervisors, drivers
13. Conduct community IEC sessions.	×	×	×	×	×	×	×	×	×	×	×	Supervisors, distributors
14. Set personal goals for the distributors.	×	×	×	×	×	×	×	×	×	×	×	Supervisors
15. Register new users.	×	×	×	×	×	×	×	×	×	×	×	Distributors
16. Provide information about family planning and contraceptives to 4000 new users, broken down as follows:												Distributors
–320 new users over months 2–3;	×	×										
–640 new users over months 4–6;			×	×	×							
–1040 new users over months 7–9;						×	×	×				
–2000 new users over months 10–12.									×	×	×	

Activity or task	Monthly activity schedule												Personnel responsible
	1	2	3	4	5	6	7	8	9	10	11	12	
17. Maintain a logbook of users, visits, methods distributed and referrals made.		×	×	×	×	×	×	×	×	×	×	×	Distributors
18. Collect the logbook data and prepare monthly reports for the coordinators.		×	×	×	×	×	×	×	×	×	×	×	Supervisors
19. Analyse the monthly reports.		×	×	×	×	×	×	×	×	×	×	×	Coordinators
20. Hold monthly staff meetings with the field supervisors.		×	×	×	×	×	×	×	×	×	×	×	Coordinators
21. Provide technical assistance to the distributors as required.		×	×	×	×	×	×	×	×	×	×	×	Supervisors
22. Identify the distributors in need of refresher training.			×				×				×		Supervisors, coordinators
23. Conduct refresher training.				×				×				×	Trainer, supervisors
24. Prepare bi-annual progress reports and submit them to the programme director.						×						×	Coordinators
25. Review and approve the bi-annual reports.						×						×	Director
26. Prepare bi-annual financial reports.						×						×	Accountant

	Activity				Responsibility
27.	Submit the progress and financial reports to the board of directors of the organization for review.			×	Director
28.	Convene the advisory team and review the progress made towards the objectives of the programme.	×	×		Director
29.	Evaluate the programme.	×			Evaluation team
30.	Study the findings and recommendations of the evaluation.		×		Advisory team
31.	Plan the objectives, activities and budget for the following year.		×		Advisory team

123

Annex 5. Sources of contraceptives for family planning programmes

Canadian International Development Agency (CIDA)
Place du Centre
200 Promenade du Portage
Hull, Quebec
K1A 0G4
Canada

Family Planning International Assistance (FPIA)
810 Seventh Avenue
New York, NY 10019
USA

International Planned Parenthood Federation (IPPF)
Regent's College
Inner Circle
Regent's Park
London NW1 4NS
England

Japan International Cooperation Agency (JICA)
2-1, Nishi-Shinjuku
Shinjuku-ku
Tokyo
Japan

Overseas Development Administration (ODA)
Health and Population Division
94 Victoria Street
London SW1A 2NS
England

Swedish International Development Authority (SIDA)
Birgerfarlsgatan 61
10525 Stockholm
Sweden

United Nations Population Fund (UNFPA)
Programme and Technical Division
220 East 42nd Street
New York, NY 10017
USA

United States Agency for International Development (USAID)
Office of Population
Department of State, Room 720 SA-18
Washington, DC 20523
USA

Annex 6. Sources of technical assistance for CBD programmes

Family Planning International Assistance (FPIA)
810 Seventh Avenue
New York, NY 10019
USA

International Planned Parenthood Federation (IPPF)
Regent's College
Inner Circle
Regent's Park
London NW1 4NS
England

Population Services International
Suite 1520
120 East 56th Street
New York, NY 10022
USA

Program for Appropriate Technology in Health (PATH)
4 Nickerson Street
Seattle, WA 98109
USA

United Nations Population Fund (UNFPA)
Programme and Technical Division
220 East 42nd Street
New York, NY 10017
USA

United States Agency for International Development (USAID)
Office of Population
Department of State, Room 720 SA-18
Washington, DC 20523
USA

World Health Organization
20 Avenue Appia
1211 Geneva 27
Switzerland

World Neighbors
5116 North Portland
Oklahoma City, OK 73112
USA

Annex 7. Sources of information materials for family planning programmes

Sources of general information

Fundación Mexicana para la Planeación Familiar (MEXFAM)
Juarez 208
Tlalpan
14000 Mexico, D.F.
Mexico

International Clearinghouse on Adolescent Fertility
The Center for Population Options
1012 14th Street NW, Suite 1200
Washington, DC 20005
USA

International Council on the Management of Population Programmes (ICOMP)
Rs 141, Jalan Dahlia, Taman Uda Jaya
6800 Ampang
Kuala Lumpur
Malaysia

International Federation for Family Health
Jalan Makmur 24
Bandung 40161
Indonesia

International Planned Parenthood Federation (IPPF)
Regent's College
Inner Circle
Regent's Park
London NW1 4NS
England

The Pathfinder Fund
9 Galen Street
Watertown, MA 02172
USA

Planned Parenthood Federation of America
Publication Department
810 Seventh Avenue
New York, NY 10019
USA

Population Communication Services (PCS)
The Johns Hopkins University
School of Hygiene and Public Health
Center for Communication Programs
527 St Paul Place
Baltimore, MD 21202
USA

Program for International Training in Health (INTRAH)
University of North Carolina
208 North Columbia Street (344A)
Chapel Hill, NC 27514
USA

United Nations Children's Fund (UNICEF)
Division of Information and Public Affairs
UNICEF House
3 United Nations Plaza
New York, NY 10017
USA

Division of Communications and Information
Palais des Nations
1211 Geneva 10
Switzerland

**United Nations Development Programme (UNDP) Asia
and Pacific Programme for Development Training and
Communication Planning**
5th floor, Bonifacio Building
University of Life
Meralco Avenue
Pasig, Metro Manila
Philippines

United Nations Population Fund (UNFPA)
220 East 42nd Street
New York, NY 10017
USA

In many countries, contact may be made directly through the UNFPA representative.

World Health Organization
20 Avenue Appia
1211 Geneva 27
Switzerland

Sources of information materials on AIDS

National AIDS Information Clearinghouse
P.O. Box 6003
Rockville, MD 20850
USA

WHO Global Programme on AIDS
AIDS Health Promotion Resource Centre
World Health Organization
20 Avenue Appia
1211 Geneva 27
Switzerland

WHO|UNESCO AIDS Centre
UNESCO Principal Regional Office for Asia and the Pacific
920 Sukhumvit Road
P.O. Box 967
Prakanong
Bangkok 10110
Thailand

Annex 8. Model budget for a CBD programme

The form overleaf is intended as a guide for preparing a budget for a CBD programme. A blank budget form is also provided for copying. The budget should include all the anticipated costs associated with the activities or tasks outlined in the workplans (see Annex 4), which should be assigned to their appropriate categories, as indicated here.

The budget described here is for a hypothetical CBD programme that required one director working quarter-time, two secretaries and two drivers working half-time, and two coordinators, 10 supervisors and 200 distributors working full-time. The supervisors were recruited after one month, while the distributors were recruited over a 12-month period. The costs (in local currency or "LC") associated with the programme are assigned to different categories such as salaries, travel and per diem, and equipment and supplies. These costs are then further divided according to the source of funds, which may be the Ministry of Health, sponsors (e.g. donor agencies) or client fees.

Title of programme: <u>Provincial CBD pilot project</u>   Page: <u>1</u> of <u>3</u>
Budget for period: <u>01/01/92</u> to <u>31/12/92</u>

Detailed budget	Sources of funds (in LC)		
	Ministry of Health	Sponsors	Client fees
I. Salaries			
Director (quarter-time): LC1000 × 12 months × 25% = LC3000	2 000		1 000
Coordinators (2 full-time): 2 × LC800 × 12 months = LC19 200	17 200		2 000
Supervisors (10 full-time): 10 × LC500 × 11 months = LC55 000		55 000	
Secretaries (2 half-time): 2 × LC500 × 12 months × 50% = LC6000	5 000		1 000
Drivers (2 half-time): 2 × LC350 × 12 months × 50% = LC4200		4 200	
Subtotal	24 200	59 200	4 000
II. Social benefits			
Employer's contribution to social programmes (equivalent to 24.6% of salaries)	5 953	14 563	984
Subtotal	5 953	14 563	984
III. Travel and per diem			
Travel:			
Coordinators, occasional trips to the field: 2 × 8 trips × LC120 per trip = LC1920	1 920		
Supervisors, travel to the central clinic for monthly staff meetings: 10 × LC40 × 11 months = LC4400	4 400		
Supervisors, transport allowances: 10 × LC10 per day × 20 days per month × 11 months = LC22 000	22 000		
Distributors, transport allowances:			
• 40 × LC5 per day × 20 days × 2 months = LC8000	8 000		
• 80 × LC5 per day × 20 days × 2 months = LC16 000	16 000		
• 140 × LC5 per day × 20 days × 4 months = LC56 000	56 000		
• 200 × LC5 per day × 20 days × 4 months = LC80 000	60 000		20 000
Distributors, trip to annual staff celebration and awards ceremony: 200 × LC40 = LC8000	8 000		

Title of programme: <u>Provincial CBD pilot project</u>   Page: <u>2</u> of <u>3</u>
Budget for period: <u>01/01/92</u> to <u>31/12/92</u>

Detailed budget	Sources of funds (in LC)		
	Ministry of Health	Sponsors	Client fees

Per diem:
Coordinators, occasional trips to the field:
  2 × 8 trips × 2 days each × LC40 per
  day = LC1280

	1 280		

Supervisors, monthly staff meetings: 10
  × 11 meetings × 1 day each × LC40
  per day = LC4400

	4 400		

Supervisors, trip to annual staff celebration
  and awards ceremony: 10 × 2 days
  × LC40 per day = LC800

	800		

Distributors, trip to annual staff celebration
  and awards ceremony: 200 × 2 days
  × LC40 per day = LC16 000

	16 000		

Subtotal	198 800	0	20 000

IV. Equipment and supplies
Slide projector, 220 V: 2 × LC390
  each = LC780

	780		

Shoulder bags, canvass with leather rein-
  forcing: 220 × LC82 each = LC18 040

	18 040		

Notebooks for supervisors and distributors
  (including 10% surplus): 231 × LC3.5
  each = LC808.5 (approx. LC809)

	809		

Laboratory coats imprinted with organization symbol: 231 × LC12 each = LC2772

	2 772		

Airtight plastic and storage boxes for contraceptives: 220 × LC18 each = LC3960

	3 960		

Easels and flipchart paper for planning and
  information activities: 4 × LC94 each
  = LC376

	376		

Ball-point pens for distributors: 120 boxes
  of 10 pens each × LC10 per box = LC1200

	1 200		

Contraceptives: calculations based on 4000
  new users using the pill (60%); foaming
  tablets (20%); foam (10%); and condoms
  (10%):
  −2400 users × 6.5 pill cycles × LC0.50 per
    cycle = LC7800

		7 800	

  − 800 users × 3 tubes of foaming tablets
    × LC0.75 per tube = LC1800

		1 800	

  − 400 users × 3 cans of foam × LC1.0 per
    can = LC1200

		1 200	

  − 400 users × 72 condoms × LC0.10 per
    condom = LC2880

		2 880	

Subtotal	27 937	13 680	0

Title of programme: <u>Provincial</u> <u>CBD</u> <u>pilot</u> <u>project</u>   Page: <u>3</u> <u>of 3</u>
Budget for period: <u>01/01/92</u> <u>to</u> <u>31/12/92</u>

Detailed budget	Sources of funds (in LC)		
	Ministry of Health	Sponsors	Client fees

V. Other direct costs

	Ministry of Health	Sponsors	Client fees
Petrol for resupply visits: 24 trips × 20 litres per trip × LC4 per litre = LC1920		1 920	
Rent for coordinators' field offices: 2 × LC100 per month × 12 months = LC2400		2 400	
Photocopying to reproduce data collection forms: 4800 copies × LC0.50 each = LC2400	2 400		
Utilities for field offices: 2 offices × LC20 per month × 12 months = LC480		480	
Communications: LC140 per month × 12 months = LC1680	1 680		
Printing of annual awards certificates for distributors: 200 certificates × LC2 each = LC400		400	
Food and supplies for annual distributors' celebration: LC234		234	
Subtotal	4 080	5 434	0
Total budget	260 970	92 877	24 984

Title of programme: _____   Page: _____ of _____

Budget for period: _____ to _____

Detailed budget	Sources of funds (in LC)		
	Ministry of Health	Sponsors	Client fees